# FOR THE LOVE OF RUNNING

## A GUIDE TO TAKING YOUR RUNNING PERFORMANCE TO THE NEXT LEVEL

STUART KREMZNER

Copyright 2020 Stuart Kremzner

ALL RIGHTS RESERVED. This book contains material protected under International and Federal Copyright Laws and Treaties. Any unauthorized reprint or use of this material is prohibited. No part of this book may be reproduced or transmitted in any form or by any means, electronic or mechanical, including photocopying, recording, or by any information storage and retrieval system, without express written permission from the author/publisher.

ISBN Paperback: 978-1-64184-367-6
ISBN ebook: 978-1-64184-368-3

To my family, my wife Bogusia who inspires me, is always encouraging me to learn, grow and excel. To my children, Robert and Konrad, who have been a joy to watch grow, and flourish. They are all an inspiration to take on new adventures.

# Table of Contents

Disclaimer ........................................... vii

Introduction ......................................... ix

Chapter 1: Training Planning: Your Road Map to Success ... 1

Chapter 2: Running Injury Prevention .................. 25

Chapter 3: The Building Blocks of Your Training Program . 57

Chapter 4: Junior-Level Runner Development ........... 80

Chapter 5: Testing and Evaluation ..................... 92

Chapter 6: Overtraining .............................. 102

Chapter 7: Regeneration Strategies for Optimizing
         Adaptation ................................. 116

Chapter 8: Competition: Putting It All Together ........ 138

Acknowledgements . . . . . . . . . . . . . . . . . . . . . . . . . . . . . . . 147
About the Author . . . . . . . . . . . . . . . . . . . . . . . . . . . . . . . . 149
References . . . . . . . . . . . . . . . . . . . . . . . . . . . . . . . . . . . . . . 151

# Disclaimer

Before starting any exercise program you must have a physician's approval and complete physical to engage in an exercise program.

The recommendations of this book are not based on medical guidelines, hence consulting with your physician is a critical first step to engaging in any physical activity. If you have any shortness of breath, dizziness, or discomfort while exercising, stop and consult with a physician before resuming any physical activity.

All forms of exercise have risks. When you are embarking on an exercise training program you are taking full responsibility for the outcomes and risks inherent in this process. This book is intended to be a guide for runners who are looking for general advice on how to train systematically with more structure.

# Introduction

I have to admit, running did not come easy to me. Like many runners my path was fraught with trial and error training, occasional improvement in performance interspersed with injury. My biggest gains came in graduate school with fantastic coaching from Chris Mackala (Track coach at University of Montana), a science based periodized training program and focus on running technique. After a couple months running became effortless, enjoyable, and most importantly injury free. After a year I was running the fastest I ever had, going from a middle pack runner to getting on the first page of the results. After many years of coaching athletes at all levels, I wanted to put the ideas on paper so other runners could develop the same love of running and make the progress they were destined to achieve.

Running is a wonderful blend of human performance, technique, and training. At the center of it all—and most importantly—is the athlete. Without well planned training, the most talented and fit athletes can be sidelined with chronic injuries.

Running is as much a lifestyle as it is a sport. What makes the sport so special to me is the combination of being outside and the feeling of flow when running on the trails, or the smell of the track on the first warm days of Spring. Few activities leave me as mentally rejuvenated as a run. It has a meditative quality to it due to the movement and sensory experience. The training for running puts you in nature, and is a family sport that you can take your kids along for from an early age. As a coach I found running to be a great teacher of life skills, especially for kids. Even the most talented athlete will be humbled by a bad race day! We all experience failures, but also success when things start to really click.

The goal of this book is to provide a general plan so coaches and athletes will have the most basic tools to develop their knowledge and athletic talent. The book is organized to present the building blocks of training. This is how I approach the development of athletes and the thought process to execute a training plan.

A secondary goal of this book is to put years of knowledge and coaching success into a framework for any level runner to improve their fitness and reach a higher level of performance. This is intended to be a guide, not the last word for running fitness development. Athletic development is based on science; however, there is an element of art when it comes to the implementation. This is where so many coaches debate about what the "best training" is for an athlete. Every athlete is a unique organism, and top coaches must have a mastery of science, sports training theory, and applied experience to create a training program that works best for an individual athlete. One size does not fit all. I hope this general framework will give the reader the basic tools to guide their training development decisions.

As a coach, my ultimate goal for every athlete is for them to cultivate their ability to be an active participant in the training development process. It's so vital they gain the necessary knowledge and skills needed for advancement. The more an athlete knows, the more they grow! The whole system will work more effectively, and hopefully performance gains will happen faster.

Another point to mention is this is in no way a substitute for a well-qualified coach. Sports training is still a field where there is very little standardization of qualifications, hence there are many "experts" in the field without any formal education in sports training. There are literally hundreds of fitness certifications (including sport governing body certifications), most of which require no previous educational experience to sit for an exam. As a result, there are a great deal of inaccurate and non-science-based theories utilized to train athletes in the US.

As an exercise physiologist and coach, I've spent years learning how to develop athletes. This is a lifelong endeavor. As our understanding of human physiology, biomechanics, applied physiology, and human adaptation continues to evolve, as does the sport and equipment. The knowledge and information I will be sharing is based upon science (most importantly) and experience. The format is user-friendly, and may sacrifice a bit from the empirical scientific side of things, but to cover the science of any one topic can easily turn into several books!

The book also does not go into great depth with regards to improving strength, speed, and power. These areas will be covered in a second companion book on advanced training concepts.

## Some Endurance Physiology Basics

To put the applied training concepts below into context, it is important to understand some of the very basics of physiology.

If you really want to learn physiology in detail, your best bet is to read some of the following resources.

McArdle, W. D., Katch, F. I., & Katch, V. L. (2010). *Exercise physiology: Nutrition, energy, and human performance.* Lippincott Williams & Wilkins.

Kurtz, T. (1991). *Science of Sports Training.* Island Pond, VT: Stadion Publishing Company.

Every year new basic research into how the human body works has an impact on how we most effectively train and develop athletes. The three main components that elevate our capacity to run fast are:

- Maximal oxygen uptake (VO2 max)

- Lactate threshold (or anaerobic threshold)

- Work efficiency

Running is an endurance sport: the more oxygen we can get to our muscles, the faster we can run. VO2 max has been the gold standard by which we measure runners, but what makes a runner fast is a combination of the above components. If you have a big motor but poor efficiency, a less aerobically-gifted runner will be superior. Similarly, if you have a big motor but a low lactate threshold, then someone with a smaller motor and higher lactate tolerance can be faster. By making training efficient, we can incorporate all three components and increase our ability to run fast.

Maximal oxygen uptake (VO2 max) is a measure of maximal aerobic work capacity, which is driven by many sub-components within the body. One of the main components is cardiac output (stroke volume x HR). When we measure this we often tag it to a percentage of maximal heart rate.

Lactate threshold (or anaerobic threshold) is where the body is producing more lactate than it has the capability to buffer. Lactate is a product of anaerobic metabolism; when our bodies produce more then we can buffer our muscles, and motor neurons start to fatigue. At high levels our muscles will cramp. We produce lactate at all intensities of exercise, however, at higher intensities we are utilizing energy systems that produce more lactate. Once we are at a workload that is producing more lactate than we can buffer (lactate threshold) we have a finite amount of time at that work intensity. That being said, our bodies can adapt to buffer higher lactate levels and thus function more effectively. Most mere mortals start to hit their lactate threshold at 4 mmol/L of lactate. World-class runners are racing at levels of 12-16 mmol/L. I like to call this one of the wild cards of performance development because even if you may not have a high VO2 max, through focused training, you may develop the ability to work at a much higher capacity.

Work efficiency is the energy cost of running per meter, or as the steady state VO2 at a standard velocity (Karlsen and Aalberg, 2002). This has sub-components of technical efficiency, neuromuscular efficiency, muscle elasticity, and power output—all of which work synergistically. For most junior and master-level athletes, this is an area that has a great deal of room for expansion—mainly due to these athlete groups frequently not having full optimization of the components. This is another wildcard of athletic performance. I remember in my early running races having runners in their 40s passing me just off of technical efficiency alone! While I was struggling they would fluidly pass me despite my strongest physical efforts in my early 20s.

All of these components together, in different proportions for different athletes, are the physiological foundation of runner development.

So if you have 200 to 400 hours a year to train, where do you start and what is most important to put your time into? The forthcoming chapters will help guide you in these decisions so you can start to craft a training plan that will help you make faster gains in your running!

# 1

# Training Planning: Your Road Map to Success

Training planning is the optimal way to achieve consistent, predictable gains in athlete development. A professor of mine Lew Curry, used to say "Everyone needs a road map...if you have a map for Boston and you are in New York, you're in a heap of crap!" This basically sums up your training program. If you don't know where you are, how do you know

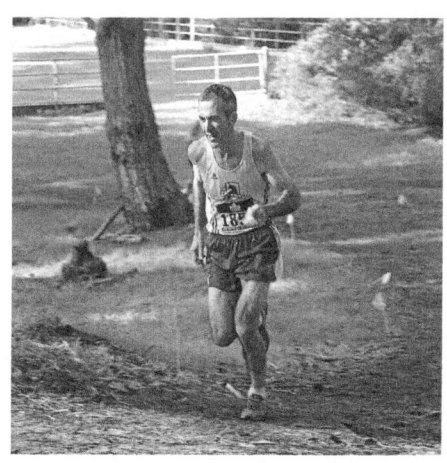

Peter Hammer on his way to 12th place in 2015 XC National Championships (Courtesy of Peter Hammer)

which way to get there? Start with obtaining a baseline evaluation of your fitness and use this to set goals and develop a good training plan, which is the map you need to achieve your performance goals. Whether you are a once a year 5k runner or national team, this is your map to success. Without a plan, achievement of goals is unpredictable and inefficient. What is your fitness level now? And how do you get to where you want to go?

The plan is where art and science are blended into an organized framework. Without it, it's difficult to determine what does and doesn't work. Without it, how do you continue to improve and innovate? The plan does not need to be complex, just organized with systematic increases in training loads interspersed with rest phases. It is ideal to have a general overview of your plan mapped out, and then fill in details based on your progress two weeks to a month in advance. That way you don't lose many hours of planning six months out when things don't go as predicted! As an athlete's abilities and level of sport mastery increase, so does the complexity and level of individualization of the training plan. This chapter will cover the basics of training plan development.

## Evaluation

For starters, you will need to assess your current fitness level, set realistic performance goals, and expand your training plan to achieve those performance goals.

Without a good evaluation you won't know if you're in Boston, New York, or Fairbanks for that matter. First and foremost you need to evaluate where you are, get an accurate baseline/assessment of what your strengths and weaknesses are; technique, endurance, ability to run at a high threshold, strength, power, speed, and most importantly injury resistance. The chapter on evaluation covers these tests and others in great detail. This is critical data for fine-tuning your training. From here you need to plan your trip and get your maps.

For running fitness aerobic tests 1000m and 3000m are good since they are standardized tests that you can use to compare yourself with others. In addition to this it's important to have your muscle function/strength and flexibility evaluated with an Original Strength or Functional Movement Screen, (FMS). This takes into account injury risk factors, muscle balance, and core strength. Lastly lactate threshold—tests need to be done. Lactate testing is best recommended for high school and master-level runners, ideally a few times a year. When you do this and your 1000/3000m test, wear a heart rate monitor to get data on speed, heart rate (HR), and average heart rate.

## Training Logs

Training logs are an important step in understanding and tracking the efficacy of your training. This does not need to be an unwieldy process, especially given the data management systems heart rate monitors have. Key data to record on a daily basis include resting HR, a subjective rating of how you feel (1–10 scale from 1- can't get out to bed to 10- I will win a gold medal today), what kind of workout you did, and how you felt doing it. You can integrate this data with your online training recording, spreadsheet, or even on a calendar. This data is critical to understand what is and isn't working with your training plan. It also allows you to see if you are starting to overtrain or are in the early stages of getting sick. Your resting heart rate is a very effective indicator of your adaptation to the training load. An increase of 10% for more than a few days should be a red flag that you are overreaching, not recovering, or getting sick.

## Periodization-The Path to Continuous Improvement

To get the most out of your training is not black magic. It requires specific, individualized goals and consistent, training planning. The key to this is periodization of training which is a step-wise organized training structure, where each week is a step to a higher level of fitness and performance. Periodization is a systematic means of structuring training elements (endurance, speed, strength, technique, and power), intensities, and loads over a 12 month period. (Fig. 1).

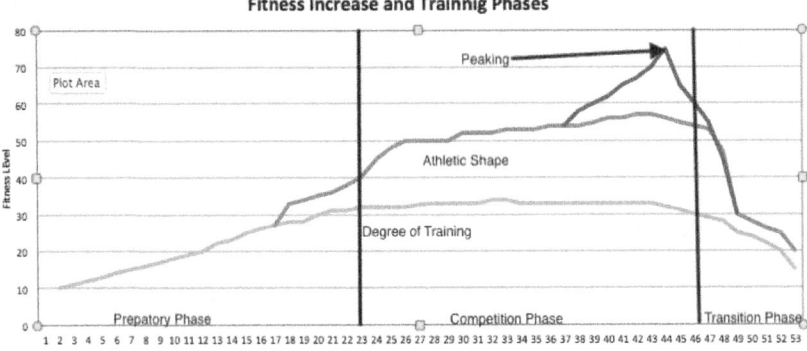

*Fig. 1: Yearly training periodization structure (adapted from Bompa, 1999)*

The conceptual framework of periodization was developed by Tudor Bompa, who revolutionized sports training theory with his book Theory and Methodology of Training (1984). Periodized training plans are usually subdivided into three distinct sub phases, Prepatory, Competition, and Transition. Each of these phases can have sub-phases. The length of these phases varies based upon the individual athlete's needs. Elite athletes tend to have longer competitive seasons whereas a beginner runner may have a competition season lasting one to two months. Generally speaking each major phase is about 3-4 months long, with the transition phase lasting about one month.

The underlying concept of periodization is; the body adapts and improves with physical stress. When the training loads (stress) is systematically varied to increase then decreased to allow regeneration our physiological capability improves, and there is an overall increase in performance. Many runners go out and run the same pace, similar distance week after week. With little structured training load changes, performance gains are minimal. Most runners will peak and plateau in 6 weeks using this system, which is what we often see at the high school level. With periodization performance gains are consistent, sometimes exceptional if the athlete has not been over-training.

Each major period has specific goals and is a step towards a consistently higher level of fitness/performance. The training year is sub-divided into progressively smaller segments, macrocycles (month long), then microcycles (week) long training segments.

**The Prepatory Phase** is structured to develop the athlete's training base. This is a time to develop the training foundation, address injury risk factors and integrate new technique. For running this is focused on developing endurance, strength, and mobility base. zThis phase can be subdivided into two sub-phases, General Preparation and Specific Preparation with progressively more focused goals. This is more relevant for intermediate to advanced level athletes. When we look at physiological development this base phase is critical fro developing the fundamental architecture for endurance sport. This is the time for those longer runs-long-steady-distance (LSD) or hikes to develop the aerobic base. These physiological changes of increasing capillarization of muscle tissue, developing stroke volume of the heart, increasing aerobic/anaerobic substrates and muscle cell mitochondrial density, take years to develop. As I have always said to the High School cross country runners I coach, their time for development is in the Spring and Summer, by the time Fall arrives their fitness is in the bank. They developed their endurance capabilities over the preceding 5 months (or not). If not, the competitive season is not the time to be putting in big miles. At that point the most important abilities to train are aerobic threshold, power, technique and speed.

## Beginnner Level Goals

- Conduct evaluation and testing, assess baseline fitness
- Set performance goals
- Develop technique through ABC drills
- Develop core strength and mobility
- Develop endurance base

## Intermediate to Advanced Level Goals

- Conduct evaluation and testing assess baseline fitness
- Set performance goals
- Develop running technique
- Develop endurance base
- Maintain peak aerobic fitness
- Develop strength and power base for more advanced speed and power training

**The Competition Phase** has two sub phases- Pre-Competition and Competition. The goal of the pre-competition phase is focused on increasing the specificity of training for the runner's main distance event. This is the time where higher levels of fitness are developed, through increased speed, interval, and power training. For marathon runners this is also the time higher volume weeks with high mileage can be put in. In this phase intensity (interval, speed and power) sessions will be increased to 3 or more sessions per week. There will also be more (1-2 per month) micro-cycles with a power and speed focus.

When the athlete enters the competition phase the primary goal is to put all the pieces together for optimal competitive fitness. In this phase the intensity of interval, speed, and power training is increased, overall volume of training will be decreased in order to allow full recovery, supercompensation and to be fresh for competitions. Early season competitions are an opportunity to have feedback to fine tune training, and pre-competition routines. I always like to tell the athletes I coach that the first few races do not matter. It is a time to try new things, test new pacing strategies and figure out what needs to be adjusted in your training to peak for the most important races later in the season. I don't like to read too much into early season results, as often athletes are transitioning from higher training hours/intensity. For individual high school runners this is the time they and the coach are figuring out the optimal balance of training, outside life stressors and how it is impacting recovery.

The competition phase has the focus of decreasing training volume and developing peak fitness in preparation for your most important competitions. In this stage you continue to maintain your endurance base, with 1-2 easy longer workouts a week, however the goal is not to develop endurance, this was done in earlier phases and the focus of fitness is on higher level capabilities lactate tolerance, maximum strength and speed endurance.

**Beginner Level Goals-** Precompetition

- Determine optimal training volume and intensity
- Develop race pace fitness
- Learn what types of intensity training worked best

**Competition**
Develop an effective pre-race routine
Learn optimal race pacing

**Intermediate to Advanced Level Goals-** Precompetition

Develop maximal aerobic capacity, anaerobic capacity and peak lactate tolerance
Develop speed and power and maximum strength
Develop Speed, maximum strength and speed endurance

**Competition**
Develop maximal aerobic capacity, anaerobic capacity and peak lactate tolerance
Develop speed and ability to change gears/pace quickly
Develop lactate tolerance, maximum strength, anaerobic capacity, and speed endurance to higher capacities, with decreased rest

**The Transition Phase** is a month long period just after the last competition with the focus of mental and physical regeneration. There should be a gradual decrease in training volume and more rapid decrease in training intensity volume. The gradual decrease in volume is important as rapid sustained decreases in training volume can result in changes mood with depression. The mode of training activity should be varied more as well to allow muscles to recover and to get the athlete refreshed. Runners can change to Nordic skiing, swimming or cycling to switch things up. If possible even have a change in environment or for master's athletes this is an ideal time for family vacation. Mentally it is important to have a break, then take some time to reflect on the season and start setting goals for the forthcoming year. Physiologically this time off allows all the systems of the body to replenish as well.

**Beginner and Advanced Level Goals**
Decrease training volume and intensity
Cross-train in different activities such as Nordic skiing, swimming, or cycling
Vacation and let body recover
Assess season training success and develop goals for improvement

Each of these primary periods consists of macrocycles which have specific fitness sub goals (increase endurance, maximal aerobic capacity, speed, strength, technique and power) for the specific phase.

**Macrocycles**
Macrocycles are one-month time periods built into the multi-month preparatory, competition, and transition phases. Each macrocycle has specific goals and structures, with the focus on developing peak fitness for your competition season. For most runners the majority of the training volume will be during the preparatory and pre-competition phases. It used to be the primary focus of these phases was lots of hours doing long, slow distance, then move to more intensity in the pre-competition and competition phases. We found, however, that this neglected many of the other key building blocks of running fitness (lactate threshold, strength, power, and speed) that could assist with making us fast. When we cycled and trained all of these abilities throughout the year, fitness and performance increased more rapidly.

Each macrocycle should have 1-2 performance evaluation sessions such as a time trial or lactate test to determine if the goals of the macrocycle were achieved. This is a learning process; it allows the athlete and coach to see if the training stimulus and structure had the desired effect. Athletes can have strong responses to some types of training and this will give the athlete/coach insight into how this athlete's body works. From there it also allows you to plan future macrocycles. For example if the coach added in lower body power training with an increased focus on strength and plyometrics and the runner's 3000m time decreased 15% that would be strong evidence that the athlete would benefit from more, or an advancement of power training in future training phases.

The loading of each phase is an individualized process, and will require some trial and error to determine what works best for you. Chart 1 shows a step-wise progression of training volume/intensity, where there is a training load increase for 3 consecutive weeks followed by a rest week. Exercise physiologists have studied this a great deal and established guidelines from which to build a program to optimize adaptation.

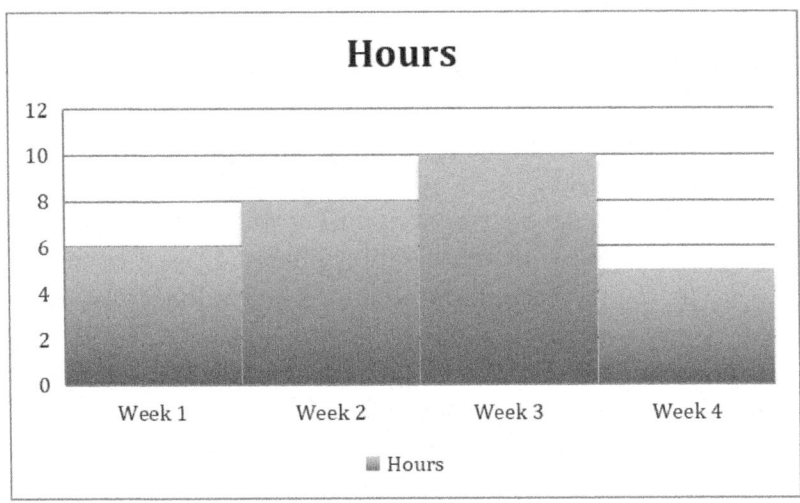

Chart 1

However, not all athletes adapt optimally to this type of loading cycle. Some have stronger adaptations to a loading sequence like in chart 2 where there are two consecutive higher load weeks followed by an easier week. This could be similar to a training camp loading cycle.

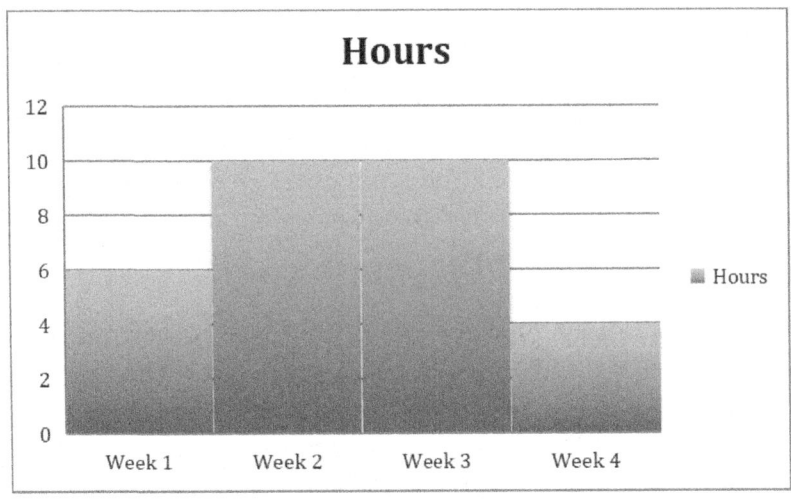

Chart 2

Lastly a progression as illustrated in chart 3 is an hard-easy-hard-easy loading progression. This sometimes works better for athletes that have lots of additional stress due to work, school, or family, that can impair regeneration, hence the regeneration has to be built more aggressively into the macrocycle training design.

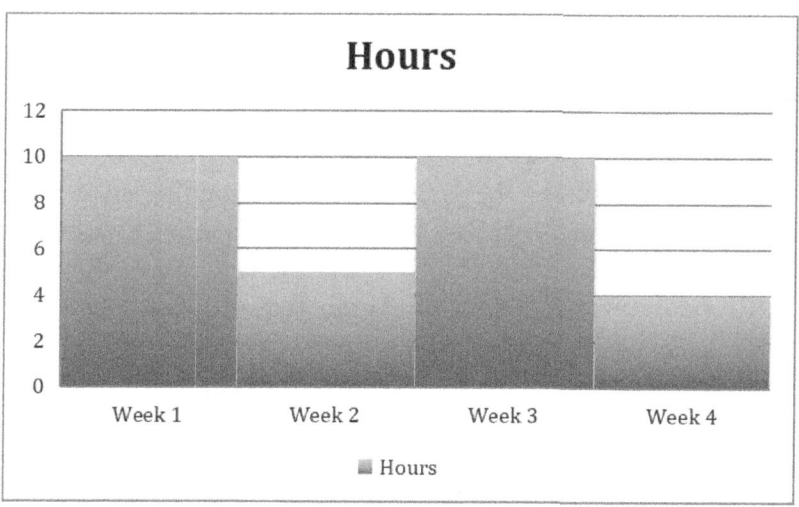

Chart 3

Different athletes respond better to different loading cycles. An alternate format is to have an increased training load for the first two weeks followed by one to two weeks of easy distance and recovery training, then repeating this cycle for one to two macrocycles. There are many ways to structure this loading; much depends upon the individual's adaptation ability, schedule, and training goals. For example, when I was a student I found a 3 week loading cycle with rest week was ideal. However in the Summer when I would have 1-2 week long camps , where all I had to do was eat, sleep and train, I found two consecutive loading weeks stimulated a supercompensation, where my performance jumped up significantly 2 weeks after the camp. Now that I am a masters athlete, I find the stepwise progression works well most of the time, but some weeks where work is very busy and regeneration is compromised I have to resort to a hard-easy-hard loading cycle to not over train. For runners new to periodized training start with a step-wise progression, but don't be afraid to mix things up and try some heavier training weeks with the expectation that you may be over-trained in the short-term. Just make sure you vary the mode (running, cycling, swimming, etc.) so you do not sustain any over-use injuries.

Macrocycle Goals are developed based on the training phase goals. I always start with an overall plan for the year. First with planning the dates of major races for my competitive season, from there I work backwards knowing my Competitive season will be 3 months long, then my Pre-competition phase will be 3 months long, Prepatory phase will then be 5 months. From there I plan general goals for each phase, and then general goals of my 12 Macrocycles, with the expectation that a month out these may change based upon my progress and what I learned worked well and didn't for my training. From two weeks to a month out I will then plan my microcycles for the given macrocycle.

**Microcycles**

Macrocycles are broken down into even smaller segments of a month, called microcycles, which are seven- to ten-day time periods. The goal of each microcycle is to be a smaller step contributing to the macrocyle goals. For example if your primary macrocycle goal is to develop your foundational aerobic capacity, your overall plan would be to increase your training volume each week., hence each microcyle you would increase your distance/hours (usually by 10% per week). Similar to macrocycles the weekly training structure is varied systematically as well. Beginner runners tend to do best with alternating hard-easy days, or hard-easy-easy-hard days. More advanced runners can benefit from doing two hard days in a row, followed by an easy day, such as a speed/track workout day, interval day, then a LSD day, then repeat the cycle, and have one day off at the end of the week. Each day you need specific goals of your training. You need to be thinking: 'What is the goal of today's workout?' Is it endurance, then make sure you stay in a L1-L2 (easy aerobic) training zone. If it is speed- then make sure you know your times for your intensity levels, you hit them, and rest enough between sets. Power -make sure you are well rested, and ready to give 100% effort with perfect technique. These principles are discussed in more detail below.

Training paradigms (loading cycles, interval structures, training complex design) differ dramatically for junior, beginner, developing, and elite athletes.

The training of athletes is a very individualized process since each athlete has different natural abilities, adaptation rates, and base levels of fitness/training. Different methods are used to stimulate and adapt. What works for your friend will not necessarily work for you. Training using standardized, cookie-cutter programs often found in magazines and websites will elicit sub-average results since they are often based upon a single runner's or coach's experience, not what works for *you*. This is why objective baseline testing is so critical.

For training to be effective, it has to be individualized and systematically modified over a long period of time. How do you do this with a team? Have a general plan designed and adjust it to the individual with different volumes and intensities as needed. You can still have a team train together but more advanced athletes may run 30 minutes longer, or do intervals that are longer. If you are on a circuit everyone will still be together and supporting each other, they just won't be in the same group all of the time.

When developing a training plan, the following training program design elements need to be taken into account:

- Training experience
- Level of competition
- Age/sex

- Energy system used
- Risk factors/injury history
- Sport/position
- Level of development/training base
- Dominant phase of training
- Level of competition

## Setting Your Training Zones

As the saying goes, "the devil is in the details." This is certainly the case of determining and applying your training zones to your workouts. Physiologists have quantified between five and eight distinct training zones for athletic fitness development. Levels 1–2 (L1, L2) are for aerobic development, Level 3 (L3) is for extensive tempo, just below race pace. Levels 4–5 (L4, L5) are for just below race pace and above race pace. Levels 6–8 (L6, L7, L8) are for speed development.

Most athletes, especially juniors and masters, tend to gravitate to training at a medium fast pace (generally Level 3). This faster pace makes you feel like you pushed hard and got a good workout in. The reality, however, *is this medium hard zone does not benefit your long-term fitness development.* For most athletes they will reach their peak performance in six to eight weeks, then plateau for months. The reason is the body has adapted to the training load and physiologically there is little to no adaptation to this level of training after six weeks; you could stay at the same level of performance for months or years. This is the case with many master and junior runners. The only difference with junior runners is their bodies are still maturing so they have improved performance gains from their physiological growth each year. Master-level runners do not have this additional maturational adaptation.

Physiologists have studied this for many years, and we know the real performance gains come from specific training in each training zone.

Training zones are tagged to heart rate, usually based upon a percentage of maximum heart rate, but this accuracy is highly variable by individual. The gold standard is to determine training zones through lactate testing. This should be done a minimum of once a year but ideally several times a year to adjust training zones for physiological adaptations.

## Training Zones: Based on Norwegian Olympiatoppen

**Level 1:** 90–98% aerobic physiological development of foundational aerobic capacity. Conversational pace, you can sing and exercise at this level. Lactate = 0.8–1.5, HR= 55–72%, 1–6 hours distance and recovery training.

**Level 2:** 80–90% aerobic, 10–20% anaerobic, physiological development of foundational aerobic capacity. Conversational pace, you can still comfortably talk and exercise at this level. Lactate = 1.5–2.5 , HR= 72–82%, 45 min–2 hours' time training, distance training at higher pace.

**Level 3:** 60–80% aerobic, 20–40% anaerobic, physiological development of lactate threshold, lactate metabolism. It is difficult to comfortably talk and exercise at this level. Lactate = 2.5–4.0, HR= 82–87%, 45–65 min time training, 5–25 min intervals to build capacity at lactate threshold. 1–3 minutes active rest.

**Level 4:** 40–60 % aerobic, 40–60% anaerobic, physiological development of maximal aerobic capacity. Hard to talk and exercise. Lactate = 4–6 , HR= 87–92%, 20–45 min time training, 4–6 min intervals to build lactate tolerance capacity. 1–3 minutes active rest.

**Level 5:** 10–20 % aerobic, 60–90% anaerobic, physiological, increase anaerobic capacity and to build peak lactate tolerance capacity. Very hard to talk and exercise. Lactate = 6–10 , HR= 92–97%, 15–30 min time training, 2.5–5 min intervals, 3 minutes active rest.

**Level 6:** Lactate tolerance training. 1–2 min intervals, 3–5 minutes rest.

**Level 7:** Speed development. 5–20 second intervals, 45–60 seconds training time, 2 minutes active rest.

**Level 8:** ATP development. 5–10 second intervals, 2 minutes active rest.

How much training should you be doing in each zone? How much endurance training and intensity should you be doing? Much of this can be determined by looking at your lactate curves. Different progressions and slopes of your lactate, speed, and heart rate curves will show what specific zones of training you will most benefit from. Good coaching based on this analysis can streamline your training program development, help you with these decisions, and adapt your training to your progress.

## Proportions of Training for Runners

Very simply put the saying

> **"When you go slow, go real slow,
> and when you go fast, go real fast,
> and avoid the in-between stuff
> because it makes you real slow"**

holds very true with many developing master and junior-level runners.

Very generally speaking, the percentage of endurance and intensity varies throughout the year. In our preparatory phase (spring and summer), the focus is on the endurance base. About 75–80% of our training hours will be in levels 1–2; 4–6% in L3; 6–8% in levels 4–5; and 2–10% in levels 6–8 doing strength, power, and speed work. When we shift to our pre-competition and competition phases, the endurance percentages decrease to 60–75%, and intensity levels change to 10–15% intensity in levels 4–8. These numbers vary widely based upon the runner's fitness and individual needs.

Master-level runners will tend to benefit from doing a higher percentage of L4–L8 intensity, as this addresses some of the fundamental limiting factors in their performance and is the most time-efficient method of training given their lifestyle.

As a point of comparison, below are training volumes of elite Norwegian 10k runners.

|  | Preparation Period | Pre-Competition Period | Competition Period |
|---|---|---|---|
| Total Km/Week | 161 | 167 | 148.2 |
| Zone 1 | 121 | 131.9 | 119.4 |
| Zone 2 | 20.1 | 11 | 10.2 |
| Zone 3 | 11.5 | 13.5 | 10.2 |
| Zone 4 |  |  | .5 |
| Zone 5 | 4.4 | 2.8 | 6.0 |
| Zone 6 | 4.8 |  | .9 |
| Zone 7 | 2 | 3.2 |  |

*Table 1: Elite runner annual training hour breakdown (adapted from, Enoksen, and Tjelta, 2011)*

How do you know if your training plan is working? The primary way will be reassessment of your baseline fitness testing. If you are improving times on your 1000m run, or favorite time trial course, then it's working, and time to progress your training by increasing your intensity or volume (but not both at the same time!).

## Supercompensation

Some athletes will experience a supercompensation after certain phases of training. This is an adaptation above the normal expected rate (5–10% gains over a two- to three-week period) and is indicative that this training had a very potent training effect. I found the two most potent factors for me were training camps, new forms of training complexes, and intensity block training (if done correctly!). Recovery during and immediately after each session, and the week after, must be optimal, as this is a huge factor in the supercompensation cycle.

## Periodization Specific for Master-Level

Master-level runners have more unique needs with periodization. We have a finite amount of time available to train with the competing time demands of work, family, and volunteer projects. With seven to ten hours a week available to train, periodization of volume is less of an option, however, we can be very creative and innovative in periodizing our intensity loading with interval, strength, and power training. For volume training, the adage that runners are made in the summer still holds true. With the longer days we can get a couple of months of good volume training in, then maintain our endurance through the fall with one or two days of endurance training. This requires a lot of efficiency of training. For this it's strongly recommended that your training zones are individualized through lactate testing.

For master-level runners that are younger and still working off a robust training base from college running or high-level competition in another endurance sport, adding in intensity blocks and speed power complexes each month for much of the year can be a very effective method of training.

## Catalysts to Performance

To optimize the time we have to train there are performance components that can give us a big bang for our training time.

### Intensity Training

The way we are thinking about physiology is changing, and research into a master-level athlete's physiology is deficient. What we do know is physiological endurance adaptations can also occur at higher levels of intensity, where we originally thought this only occurred with high volume at low intensities. For master-level runners this is an area wide open for exploration.

In my training of diverse athletes over the years I have been surprised at the aerobic fitness of athletes that come from speed-power backgrounds that spent a great deal of time training at their lactate threshold or much higher. When we look at the trends in other endurance sports, such as marathon running, many of the fastest athletes now are starting with an 800m–1500m competitive base then adding in the endurance abilities. This can be very effective, as these runners have perfected their running efficiency at high speeds. Given this foundation, if the athlete develops their endurance base, this high running speed will be a dominant neuromuscular skill that will optimize the endurance capability. I believe that an increased proportion of speed and power training holds an untapped potential for many master and junior-level runners.

### Strength, Power, and Speed Training

This area is one of the most unexplored in terms of research and application to endurance athletes, however, the limited research studies have been very positive. If we can improve our neuromuscular efficiency we will improve our running efficiency.

**Strength and Power** training are catalysts to achieving this. With increased force output we not only can have improvement in our endurance capacity (i.e., it takes less energy to achieve the same workload), it also allows us to develop higher amounts of force in general through the training of elastic qualities of our muscles and tendons by producing even higher amounts of force. Numerous studies have found excellent improvements that generalize over to running endurance performance. These neuromuscular improvements will generalize over to increased running efficiency. Hoff et al. (1999) found maximal strength training in Nordic skiers over nine weeks increased time to exhaustion by 60%. For endurance runners Storen (2008) found strength training increased running efficiency by 5% over eight weeks. Heggelund (2013) found maximal strength training increased work economy by 31%, and rate of force development was increased by 13.7%. In addition Saunders et al. (2006) found that a nine week plyometric program increased running efficiency by 4.1% at higher running speeds in elite runners. Lastly Paavolainen et al. (1999) found explosive strength decreased 5k times in runners by about 1 minute and ground force reaction times decreased by 8% after a 9 week strength and power training program.

**Speed Training** is the next layer of developing an improvement in running performance. By speed training I am referring to structured higher intensity running over distances of 500m or less. Research by Faiss et al. (2015) found that repeated sprint training increased runners' power output by 11% over six sessions (each consisting of four sets of five 10-s sprints, with 20-s intervals of recovery). Additional research has shown speed training to be highly effective in improving endurance performance, (Skovaard, et al. 2018), Lastly Iaia & Bangsbo (2010), did a review of research and found a 3-15% improvement in endurance performance (depending on protocol and length of time) with different types of speed training. For a 21 minute 5k this would be more than 2 minute decrease in time! That is not too bad for a mid level runner doing speed training over 2-4 weeks!

The goal of speed training is threefold:

- To increases one's tolerance and buffering capacity of high levels of lactate.
- To increase limb velocity and develop increased force output through increased power output and improve the force elasticity properties of muscle/tendon tissues.
- To improve peak velocity and efficiency at higher running speeds (i.e., stimulate a neuromuscular adaptation that will generalize over to improving race pace).

There is no doubt that this can yield a significant improvement in endurance running performance. Through my own personal training and coaching experiences I have found speed training to be very effective in developing a supercompensation that improved 5k and 10k running times, far more effectively than 3-4 years of high volume endurance training. Adding in track workouts also is a nice way to switch up the regular training routine, not to mention getting a big bang for your training effort.

Implementation of more detailed strength, power, and speed exercises will be covered in the following chapter.

**Volume Blocks and Maintenance**

Master-level runners often don't have the flexibility of a schedule to consistently get those long, easy workouts in. With family commitments and lots of extra side projects, plans for that six-hour hike or bike ride often get shifted to the back burner to shuttle kids to the soccer game or have family time.

One way to build your endurance fitness is to have one microcycle a month with training volume as the focus. In this week you could get 1–2 easy (level 1–2) high-volume weekend days in (2–4+ hours), then one session mid-week of 1.5–2 hours. This could provide a total L1 and L2 weekly volume of 5.5–12 hours. The following weeks you would then just need one Level 1 active rest day of 1–1.5 hours of easy volume then another day of 2–3 hours in Level 1–2 to maintain your base.

Another option is during weeks you have vacation or a lighter schedule, add in a high volume or "mini-camp" week then progress consecutive weeks as shown above. This type of training structure is a way to progressively increase and maintain your endurance base. If your focus is on marathon racing, this structure is critical to your success. If your racing focus is primarily 10–15k races then you may be able to get away with overall lower training volumes. The best time of the year to increase your training volume is in the summer and fall. When you are in the pre-competition phase (November and December), you will be shifting your focus to higher intensity training, and in your competition phase focus on high-quality intensity, racing, and staying well-recovered.

## General Rules for All Ages

1. Training volume increases should be done consistently and structured such that volume increases are a gradual 5–10% increase per week/month, otherwise overtraining can result.

2. Intensity levels can increase 3–6% over a four-week period.

3. You can only focus on training 1–2 new abilities (speed, strength, aerobic threshold training, endurance, etc.) over a microcycle otherwise your body will not adapt as efficiently.

4. In order to develop an biomotor ability (speed, for example) you need to train it at least twice per week.

5. For anaerobic threshold development, 1–2 interval sessions per week maintains fitness, 3 increases aerobic capacity.

6. When you go slow, go very slow and when you go fast, go fast. The in-between stuff does not teach your body much.

7. Train to race, don't race to train.

8. Every workout needs to have a specific purpose and goal. This purpose must fit in synergistically with the microcycle plan.

9. Keep a training log documenting how you feel and what you did for training.

10. **Most important:** keep your training fun!

## Plan Development

Given the above information, you have the necessary ingredients to develop your program. As a coach it is important to teach your athletes to have a strong understanding of their training planning. This will help the athlete avoid too much trial and error.

When you are putting together your map start with these key points:

1) Start your plan with figuring out which races you are peaking for, then work backwards with the general outline.

2) Don't get too detailed in the long-term planning since everything may change given your adaptation rates, illness, and new information on training.

3) Plan details 7–10 days in advance based upon the way you feel and how well you have adapted.

4) For junior-level runners, use other competitive sports as base conditioning for running, but try to get two run-specific technique workouts in per week. This can be as simple as two 15-minute sessions of stride development drills, and some tempo. 5) Have two primary specific goals for each

microcycle (i.e., endurance base development and technique, anaerobic threshold training and max-strength).

With a good training plan you will progress forward and upward, with few setbacks. The most important thing is to enjoy the journey and not get too lost in the process!

# 2

# Running Injury Prevention

Over many years of coaching junior and masters runners I have seen the same recurrent injuries year after year that sideline runners for weeks to months. 65-75% of runners are injured annually (Hanlon, 1987). Think about that for a second, 3/4 of runners are sidelined with injury each year. Through my experience most of these injuries are preventable with a well-designed training program that integrates core stability, mobility, strength, and sound training principles with technical development.

Taunton et al. (2002) compiled a list of common overuse injuries suffered by runners:

- Patellofemoral pain syndrome
- iliotibial band syndrome
- plantar fasciitis
    - the above accounted for 32% of all running injuries

- meniscal injuries
- patellar tendinopathy
- Achilles tendonitis
- Shin splints
- knee/hip pain
- stress fractures

A further breakdown of the data amalgamated by Taunton revealed the following:

- Female runners accounted for almost twice the rate of Patellofemoral pain and iliotibial band syndrome cases as males.
- Male runners reported 2x as many cases of meniscus injuries and 3x as many gluteus medius injuries as their female counterparts.
- Runners in general with less than 8.5 years of experience were at a higher risk of injury as compared to those with a longer training history.

Most of the injuries mentioned have a few commonalities in their root cause. Once such commonality is over striding. Over striding while running refers to the athlete reaching or placing the foot too far out in front of the body (center of gravity) causing the foot to slam down into the ground. The result is an inefficient running stride, characterized by larger than optimal breaking forces applied to the lower body. The reasons for over striding can vary from person to person but are typically driven by mobility, stability and strength imbalance factors Souza (2016), Milner (2006), and Noren et al. (2014), (2012) Where the breaking point (injury) occurs is largely a function of individual makeup and training idiosyncrasies.

As a physiologist I have spent most of my career developing methods to prevent injury. In doing so, a fundamental understanding of the mechanisms of injury are requisite to the design of an effective training program focused on injury prevention and performance. As previously noted, most injuries are caused by fundamental imbalances of optimal mobility and stability. The dysfunctional interplay between these two essential elements of locomotion can lead to a laundry list of issues to include:

- Increased impact forces (due to overstriding)
- Altered/compensated muscle firing patterns which put additional stresses/activity on adjacent muscle groups
- Restricted range of motion of joints specifically ankle, hip and spine
- Inability to have proper body position
- Inability to balance and have dynamic stability
- Inability to transfer and manage forces generated by our muscles

"A potential driver of poor running kinematics are a lack of, or simply inefficient reflexive core stability strategies. This issue fundamentally prevents an expression of the full range of motion of the lower body. To understand this concept, an assumption is made that the human body is inherently designed to covet stability over mobility.

When the reflexes that drive the stabilizing muscles of joints crucial to locomotion - in this case we are talking about the central core - have become slow or neurally pruned (due to lack of use or previous injury) the body seems to compensate by using prime movers to stabilize the involved joint(s).

Since these muscles can not be movers and stabilizers at the same moment in time, the body will default to stability over mobility and a loss of range of motion can be noted.

Hence sub-optimal reflexive control of the core leads to compensatory movement and stability strategies in an attempt to provide the articulating limbs with a solid base of operation. The net result to the end user of said strategy is one of restricted range of motion or in a worst case scenario - pain and injury." (Shropshire, 2020)

Poor mechanics due to mobility deficiency or poor running technique in turn results in over-striding which dramatically increases the impact forces while running. All this extra pounding will result in stress related injuries such as shin splints, plantar fasciitis, and joint injuries. Injuries related to mobility and core strength deficiencies tend to be iliotibial band syndrome and gluteal medius injuries.

**What is Over-striding? How can I tell if I am over-striding?**

Over-striding is where the foot impacts the ground in front of the center of gravity. Niemelä et al. ( 2017) found that the impact (ground reaction forces) of runners over-striding at training pace are 2.5-3 times greater than the runner's body weight, with an average of 550-700 strides per mile this is an immense amount of cumulative stress on the lower extremity.

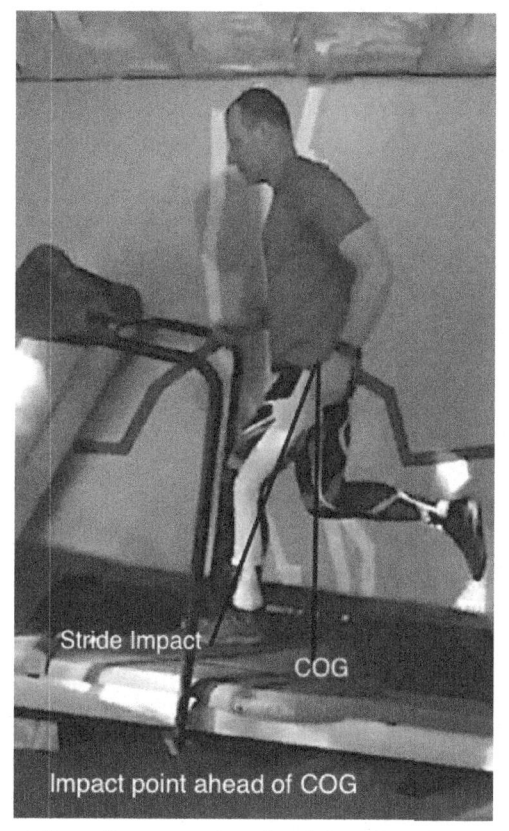

Over-striding-Impact ahead of the Center of Gravity

Lieberman et al. (2010) found that 75-80% of runners with conventional running shoes over-stride due to being rear-foot strikers. This correlates highly with close to 75% of runners being injured annually. There are multiple factors that contribute to over-striding;

- Bad running mechanics
- Impairment in ankle mobility
- Posterior pelvic tilt i.e. hips are back (due to core strength deficiency) which moves center of gravity back
- Mismatch in shoes relative to running mechanics i.e. too much heel lift in running shoe

Most runners are unaware they are over-striding, they may think the feeling of impact with each step is normal or just do not notice due to foot cushioning. The easiest way to see if you are over-striding is to have an experienced coach watch you run on a treadmill or track. A quick filming and slowing of the frames will show where your contact point is relative to your center of gravity. The other way is to listen to; your feet as they make contact with the ground or treadmill. If you notice a loud pounding or heavy slapping sound on impact - chances are you may be overstriding.

The next step is to determine the root cause of over-striding. Certainly teaching better running technique will help, however most runners have mobility or strength deficits that make it very difficult for them to achieve (and maintain for a full run) correct technique.

So where to start? The first step is a skilled evaluation to determine where your injury risk factors are. Secondly, active and regular utilization of a movement restoration program that addresses these deficiencies is paramount to success. One such system of restoration is called Original Strength. The exceedingly simple yet effective exercises and movements of Original Strength rewire the brain in such a way as to create an optimal foundation for more complex movement strategies - such as running! (Shropshire, 2020) As you are working on this foundation you can start basic stride development exercises to pattern the correct neuro-muscular firing pattern. The next step is a running biomechanics assessment by a skilled professional. This will give you feedback on any other deficits and mechanical deficiencies and steer your training towards more efficient and focused efforts. Many runners have never been taught how to run efficiently through the application of stride development drills. These drills will go a long way to help improve running efficiency and reduce running injury. These will be covered in the next section, but for now, let us dive a little deeper into what I believe are some of the root causes of these issues to begin with.

## MOBILITY AND STABILITY- THE FOUNDATION OF PERFORMANCE

The body's musculo-skeletal system (kinetic chain) mobility and stability are an interdependent foundation of all other aspects of fitness, one balances the other like a see-saw. When not fully developed (and this is the case in many elite athletes), we will see injuries, technique deficits, and minimal gains from higher- level fitness elements like strength, power, and speed. Gray Cook, in his books <u>Athletic Body in Balance</u> and <u>Movement</u>, talks of mobility as the freedom of movement of multiple muscles and joints, then stability as 'the ability to control force'.

As a coach, I would be frustrated by some athletes' inability to develop good technique (like lifting the knees when sprinting) despite countless hours spent on drills and cueing efforts.

According to Cook and other authorities on human locomotion, a potential rationale for this dilemma is actually quite simple. The athlete can't perform to standard because their body will not let them move that way due to mobility, stability, or asymmetrical deficits. For example a restriction in ankle mobility will limit the amount of lean angle in running, which in turn limits the maximal velocity one can move. Tight hip flexors/hamstrings or weak core will limit the amount of pelvic rotation one can have or maintain(i.e. the butt pushing back), which change the center of gravity, hence contributing to over-striding.

Many of us have also coached athletes who are strong, but after many hours of work they did not develop to expectation. This, too, is a symptom of a mobility/stability deficit, as any higher-level development will not be optimized with an unstable foundation. Gray refers to this as the 'Over-powered' athlete. They are strong but frequently injured. Using a car analogy - this is due to too big of a motor for too small of a suspension. Essentially their musculoskeletal system cannot effectively manage the power their primary mover muscle groups are generating.

A simple system exists to evaluate and address this: the Functional Movement Screen. Many of us have heard of Gray Cook's book <u>Athletic Body in Balance</u>, a hidden gem in its implications for developing athletes by addressing these kinetic-chain imbalances. Once we diagnose and fix kinetic-chain deficits (like core instability where an athlete has difficulty balancing on one leg, or stabilizing upper and lower body) we can progress athletes much faster.

From the time we are born, our body's musculoskeletal and nervous systems start compensating and adapting to environmental stresses, such as repetitive movement, bad posture from sitting and working on a computer for an hour a day or injuring an ankle so we lose ankle mobility and stride length. Much of the body's adaptation is in a positive manner, however as we mature our bodies are exposed to a host of repetitive stresses (and sometimes traumas) that can cumulatively cause movement restrictions and imbalances in our body's movement, stability, and strength. This will cause inefficiencies in movement and power application.

With movement restrictions, no matter how hard we try, we cannot achieve an efficient body position. This compensated body position will not allow us to run efficiently. This can be very frustrating to beginning and advanced runners alike, and very perplexing to a coach. Why can't this runner push their hips forward to get in a good body position? Why are they hunched or struggling to balance?

Coaches have runners stretch, strengthen and do planks for minutes on end, yet problems persist. In order to more effectively address this, we need to think about, evaluate and train the musculoskeletal system as an interrelated system. In this model refined by Cook and Thomas Myers, the muscles are thought of as a series of myofascial slings (a network of muscles) that extend the full length of the body. Hence what aches you have in your back can be driven by tightness in your foot or shoulder, as they are connected through the same muscular networks (myofascial slings).

Your skeletal system works in tandem with this system. Its stacked joints alternate their roles between stability and mobility. Mike Boyle explains this in depth in his article "A Joint by Joint Approach to Training". The ankle is a mobile joint, knee, a stable joint, hip mobile, lumbar (Lower) spine-stable, Thoracic spine- mobile, joints alternate mobility and stability.

| Joint | Primary Training Need |
| --- | --- |
| Ankl | mobility (particularly sagittal) |
| Knee | stability |
| Hip | mobility (multi-planar) |
| Lumbar Spine | stability |
| T-Spine | mobility |
| Gleno-humeral | stability |

So what usually happens if you lose ankle mobility due to multiple injuries or tight muscles? The mobility has to happen somewhere so it gets transferred to an adjacent joint, usually the knee, which is meant to be a stable joint. The knee does not like mobility nor is it designed to be mobile so it gets sore or even much worse injured (Patellofemoral pain syndrome, iliotibial band syndrome, meniscal injuries, patellar tendinopathy).

Trying to fix a single problem, for example hip tightness or knee pain, will not be as effective as addressing the whole system. One muscle group does not work in isolation, nor should we train it in such a manner. In order to achieve proper body position when skiing, we first need to address movement restrictions to allow it to move freely and efficiently. Cook has taken this concept to a user-friendly level and developed a system of evaluation and corrective exercises.

For example, think about how many hours per day students and adults are seated. This seemingly benign activity will cause a variety of mobility and altered muscle firing pattern dysfunctions, such as tightened hip flexors and altered glute/hamstring functioning (glute amnesia).

How does this affect a runner? From running studies we know that for each degree of anterior hip rotation we gain 2.5 centimeters of stride length. It is common with tight hip flexors to have a 5- to 10-degree deficit; think about the impact an improvement of this could have on one's overall race pace. Sitting for prolonged periods of time, with the hips flexed in the presence of poor reflexive core stability leads to over activation of the hip flexors in an attempt to compensate for an underperforming muscle synergist. In addition, if the glutes are turned off, (most likely due to a phenomenon known as reciprocal inhibition caused by their functional antagonist, the hip flexors being overactive) the hamstrings and lower back are taxed with an inordinate amount of work in creating hip extension to compensate for the now poorly functioning gluteal muscle complex. As the glutes are a major driver to the power of locomotion, the runner who suffers from this "glute amnesia" is also susceptible to a knee that is less stable, and overworked (not weak as is sometimes indicated) lower back - in the end, someone is going to be unhappy (i.e. knee or back pain, hamstring pulls).

As runners, we strive for movement efficiency and optimal power production. To achieve this we need to evaluate runner's mobility, stability and optimal muscle function. This is best achieved through an advanced Functional Movement Screen (FMS), Original Strength Screen and Assessment, or a very well done kinetic-chain physical therapy evaluation. For the coach, courses and certifications are offered by both FMS and OS to help build a better understanding of movement and how to create systems to benefit athletes with sub optimal movement patterns.

## ORIGINAL STRENGTH THE FIRST STEP FOR IMPROVED MOBILITY AND STABILITY

Like most coaches, I have been on the eternal quest to get the most out of an athlete's performance. Not all of us are born with VO2 maxes in the 80's so we need to do lots of tuning to get the most out of our motors. When a runner comes by on the course I do the quick checklist of what is holding this athlete back. More often than not I see the inability to maintain an efficient body position, as the limiting factor. The fundamental commonality between all these elements is reflexive core strength. This element is one of the most important for technical efficiency for all runners from beginner to elite to improve. Some people reading this right now are thinking "I can do a plank for 2 minutes, no problem. What do you mean I might have an unstable or un-reflexive core?" A four-point plank is static core, i.e. not reflex driven, and as such, may not be as effective of an exercise to train reflexive core stability as you think. Core strength exercises must be <u>dynamically and reflexively driven</u> to transfer over to be effective for sports performance. As taught by Tim Anderson and the staff at Original Strength….. by reflexive, we mean without conscious thought. Here is a simple example of how the core is set up to function based on reflex information. Lay on your back and simply lift your head up to look at your toes. Your abdominal wall will fire without you thinking about it. Now put your head down and lift both of your legs off the ground. Did you feel your core contract just before you lifted your legs? That is reflexive stability. Some of you might have even felt your core turn on as you began to think about lifting your head or legs. Reflexive stability/strength is also predictive strength as well. Through repeated exposures to movements (training) we are able at a subconscious level, to anticipate the movement and stability strategy necessary to accomplish the given task. When these movements involve the patterning of the gait cycle in such a way that we expose the core to stress, the brain adapts by improving the speed of the reflexes necessary to activate the muscles responsible for stability. As a result, the brain develops neural engrams (think of neural super highways) to further speed the process of reflexive stability for a given pattern of movement. If that pattern more resembles the human gait cycle - the better the brain gets at creating a reflexively stable core to support it. (Shropshire, 2020)

In 2003 Gray Cook introduced and expanded the importance of mobility and stability in the performance hierarchy. Without this solid foundation of the ability to control movement and have a full range of movement everything else we add on for fitness and performance development will not be optimal. Gray touched on the topic of "primitive patterns" of movement that has gotten much greater recognition. Tim Anderson and Geoff Neupert expanded on the concept in their book Pressing Reset. In it they describe the concept of "Resets" patterned after the neuro developmental movement sequence – the sequence of movement that infants use to develop enough core stability to stand on two feet and walk. In Original Strength Performance the Next Level – the concept was applied to the performance realm. They learned that re-setting the nervous system prior to dynamic core exercises yielded exceptional results in re-developing and maintaining efficient core strength and movement patterns. Resets are like wiping your hard-drive for your neuromuscular system, if we don't erase the dysfunctional pattern it will continue to delay development. Neurophysiologically we are born with a blueprint for optimal, efficient, movement patterns, designed to get us up on two feet and walking. This blueprint is exploited through simple sequences of breathing, head movement, rolling, and crawling. After about 4-6 years if we don't use our core the way we were designed to use it, we start to lose it. We are seeing this more and more given lifestyle changes in today's increasingly sedentary society. How many of the kids we coach are doing manual labor these days and spending hours outside running and playing? Our movement pattern's base level functioning is dictated by the dominant motor programs we use. Our bodies were designed to be up and mobile 8-10 hours a day. Put us in a chair for 6-8 hours a day (like with school kids) or a desk jockey job and we have global changes in the de-tuning and functioning of our neuro-muscular system. Primary core muscles develop dysfunctional firing patterns and weaken. Hip flexors shorten, posture changes (we get more stooped). Our core muscles stop firing optimally in their original motor program, they are not turning on at the right time or not at all. This leads to altered/decreased muscle firing sequences, compensated movement patterns, power leaks, injuries, and for many of us, decreased athletic performance.

For years as coaches and physiologists we have been focused on more speed, power, strength and endurance. However, all this work is not optimized if we don't have the fundamental ability to generate power, transfer it effectively between joints then into the ground, and have optimal mobility to use the full length of all of our muscle fibers effectively.

Reflexive core strength is the foundation of efficient all movement patterns. Hip stabilization and coordinating segmented movements between the upper and lower body is primarily mediated/controlled by our deep pelvic floor and transverse abdominal muscles. The key is to keep the core exercises dynamic and reflexive, (it is reflexes that drive the optimal functioning of the deep reflexive core). Good running technique does not consist of doing static planking for 5 minutes. The exercise needs to be dynamic, hence you need to lift an arm, leg, or both (with proper body alignment) to keep the plank reflexive. It is important to do perfect technique. It is far more effective to do perfect technique for 3 seconds vs poor technique for 30 seconds (this just keeps reinforcing the dysfunctional muscle firing pattern!)

What follows are some ideas and the very basic science behind activating and training your reflexive core. Think of this as your 'quick start' guide. For individualized/targeted training you need to have a good evaluation with a Original Strength certified coach who can develop a program that is most effective for you. At the very least this will help get you started. These exercises were developed by Tim Anderson and Geoff Neupert of Original Strength.

Before and after each exercise grab a 10-20kg weight and do a deep squat, then a toe touch. Pay attention to how it feels, range of motion, and 'snap' you have going down and coming up.

To start, you need to reset and 'overwrite' the dysfunctional movement programs in your nervous system. These exercises are called 'resets'. "Resets are the ABC's of movement. When you can put all the letters together you can begin to make words, then before you know it you can make sentences. Sentences become paragraphs and eventually masterpieces of literature! Movement is a lot like this – it starts out simple and messy and through practice becomes a thing of beauty. It starts with the resets of Original Strength." (Shropshire, 2018) ) This is achieved through systematically activating the muscle firing patterns as we developed them when we were infants/toddlers. These recruitment patterns originate in the more primitive part of our brain (brainstem, medulla oblongata pons, cerebrum) , this is the foundational center of our most basic movement patterns. Through aging, injury, dysfunctional pattern overrides (sitting 8 hours a day) these fundamental patterns are overridden by altered muscle firing patterns that are not efficient.

The fundamental resets are diaphragmatic breathing, head nods, rolling, rocking and crawling. Each exercise has a video link to view excellent technique. If your squat or toe touch feels better and you can move with more depth and ease that is a good reset for you.

It all starts with diaphragmatic breathing. Diaphragmatic breathing is critical to resetting and activating your core. The diaphragm along with the transverse abdominis and pelvic floor form the basic reflexive core. Intentional breathing using the diaphragm activates the other muscles of the reflexive core via neural and fascial connections – hence it is the gateway into the reflexive core. Head nods and rolling help reset and stimulate your ocular- vestibular system which is integrally related to developing proprioception and balance.

1-**Diaphragm Breathing** (restores muscle proprioceptive reactivity, helps you use your diaphragm which besides being a major respiratory muscle, is also a core stabilizer. Also shifts CNS from sympathetic to parasympathetic ) - Lay on stomach (or back), forehead resting on flat hands, legs extended. Belly breathe deeply in and out through your nose. Your exhale should be 2x as long as your inhale. Tongue should be pressing on the roof of your mouth just behind your teeth. On the inhale push your belly button into the ground and push it up as much as possible. Belly should always rise before shoulders. Breathe for about 2-3 mins, then flip over on your back and hold your knees up with your hands and keep focusing on the deep breaths for another 1-2 mins.
Video Link Here-Diaphragmatic Breathing in Prone - https://www.youtube.com/watch?v=nH-dpQYzvz4&feature=youtu.be

Diaphragmatic Breathing in Supine - Knees to Chest-https://www.youtube.com/watch?v=FTOXynkzeTg&feature=youtu.be

Video- https://www.youtube.com/watch?v=Qt3eYc5l8Xg

The key with all these exercises is to maintain the same tempo and depth of diaphragmatic breathing.

2- **Head nods**- lay on back arms at 45 degrees, palms up, legs extended. Have eyes look back, extend neck and head rotating to

the point where forehead is touching floor, then roll eyes down, flex your neck downward toward the sternum and lift your head off the ground to look between heels. Repeat 10x (keep the same breathing depth and rhythm).
Video Link Here- Head Nods-https://www.youtube.com/watch?v=sSLYvheWpVA&feature=youtu.be
https://www.youtube.com/watch?v=edmP-35MyW8

3- **Rolling** – There are many types of rolling variations, different types of rolls are more effective for improving various movement patterns. Start with Egg Rolls then move to Segmental Rolling.

**Egg Rolls**- Lay on your back and pull your knees up to your chest, holding them with your hands. Then, leading the movement with your eyes, look to the side and rotate your head and let the body follow. Then, look the opposite direction with the eyes, then move the head to initiate the roll. Use as little energy as possible. This should feel relaxed and easy, keep rotating your head all the way though for complete range of motion. Video Link Here-https://www.youtube.com/watch?v=LRSd2mk-U2A&feature=youtu.be

**Segmental Rolling**- there are two types of segmental rolls. One using the legs as the impetus for movement, the other using the arms.
- Lower body rolls: Begin on your back with arms comfortably resting overhead on the ground. Begin by lifting one leg toward the rib cage as far as you can. Then cross the midline of your body and simply let the weight of the leg roll you over. To roll back into a supine position, bend your knee and lift your leg off the ground and across the midline of the body. Allow the weight of the leg to roll your body over. Video Link Here-https://www.youtube.com/watch?v=F-NjQXiL4jwo&feature=youtu.be
- Upper body rolls: The same type of instruction applies here. Pick your head up, look in the direction you want to roll,

then reach your hand across the midline of the body and allow the body to roll over into a prone position. To return to the supine position, pick your head up and then your arm. Sweep the arm across the midline of your body to initiate the roll back to supine.
Video Link Here- https://www.youtube.com/watch?v=OnvM3_dKBh0&feature=youtu.be

5) **Rocking**- On hands and knees. Keep head/neck extended, rock back and flex neck, keep back in level alignment, elbows are locked out with body/neck extension and flexion. Rock slowly forward and backward maintaining breathing a diaphragmatic breathing pattern. Do 20 reps.
Video Links Here- https://www.youtube.com/watch?v=plHqt_NBH1E&feature=youtu.be
Video- https://www.youtube.com/watch?v=EEJ4ADGu1FA
https://www.youtube.com/watch?v=irEFUp3SHc4

6) **Baby Crawls**- 3x30m- Keep your head up, diaphragmatically breathe as you move. Lift a hand and the opposite knee off ground as you move forward. Allow the foot to drag along the ground . Once you can do this perfectly progress to keeping knees off the ground (about 2-3 cm, no more). Video- https://www.youtube.com/watch?v=kGIQ4szkb4c

## GETTING THE MOST OUT OF EVERY STEP STRIDE DEVELOPMENT DRILLS TO OPTIMIZE YOUR RUNNING EFFICIENCY

Every start of the season coaching masters and high school runners, I immediately get quisical looks when I start talking about stride development drills. The first response is always "that is what sprinters do, I just want to run!", or "Those are too high intensity I will get injured!" These often are the runners I see hobbling around 2 months into their season with chronic shin splints, or other lower extremity injuries. To be clear the purpose of these drills is to teach efficient mechanics with the least amount of braking forces. Who does not want to run faster and more comfortabley at the same exertion level? Yes, the mechanics that are being taught were originally developed for sprinters, but aren't they runners too? Most importantly these drills will teach you to run with correct mechanics which will prevent injuries and improve running efficiency.

Running speed is the product of two components;
Stride Length (SL) x Stride Frequency (SF)

Increase either and you run faster. Most elite runners have the same stride frequency of 84 -91 strides per minute (Daniels, 2005), Liberman et al. (2015). Which means the difference between these runner's varied pace is a factor of stride length. Liberman et al. (2015) did find that a stride frequency of 85 was optimal metabolically. It is important to understand that stride length is developed by putting more power into the ground for forward propulsion, and minimizing braking forces, **not** by reaching farther forward with the leg and impacting the ground ahead of the hip (this improper technique will lead to extensive risk of injury).

Stride development drills will teach us how to apply power into the ground correctly and efficiently to improve stride length.

The following sequence of drills will help you develop excellent running mechanics. When implemented daily into your running program you will start to see the results in the improvement of your running efficiency and reduction of injuries. Imagine improving your running stride length by 2 inches, multiply this by 10,000 strides and you will have a new PR! As with all drills, these are an exaggeration of technique to some degree, with practice like this your intrinsic motor program technique change/adaptation will be more rapid.

For starters I like to teach runners good body position. One commonality among many elite runners is that they have a 3.5 degree body lean position (Preece et al, 2016) . This body lean is from the ankles, not at the waist. This technical element is critical as it improves running efficiency and reduces the braking forces on the lower extremity which reduces LE injury.

In the 1950's a Polish track coach Gerard Mach developed a standardized set of running mechanic drills to teach runners how to optimally apply power into the ground to run faster and more efficiently. If you think of your leg more as a turning wheel (i.e. we want to keep the wheel spinning as fast as possible with the least amount of friction (braking forces) , these drills will make more sense. Mach subdivided the stride into 3 distinct phases:

**Hip Flexion /High Knee- (Skip A)-** The purpose of this drill is to teach the body the correct knee lift and starting position to deliver power into the ground. The optimal position is 90 degrees of hip flexion (past 90 degrees is not longer effective as it actually creates backward momentum). The purpose of this is two fold; Increased force production and propulsion efficiency. Imagine your foot has a hammer, the longer the swing of the hammer the more force you can put into your stride. The second benefit is it effectively unweights the rest of your body; as this knee swings rapidly up, the movement creates forward momentum. Swinging 10% of your body weight up and forward is that much less weight to push your body forward with each stride.

**Contact Phase -Clawing Action (Skip B)-** The purpose of this drill is to teach the runner where to correctly contact the ground and apply pulling force underneath the body. (Remember the hammer analogy). Over-striding is the biggest source of injury in runners.
Stand tall, squeeze butt cheeks to have optimal anterior pelvic tilt, Extend leg, dorsi-flex ankle, sweep (or claw) foot back

contacting the ground just under the hip, continue sweeping back, keeping hips in the same position (do not let them break!)

**Push-off/Extension and Recovery Phase- Butt Kick (Skip C)-** This is the extension and recovery phase of the power application. The goal of this drill is to continue pulling back (applying full power) to complete extension (without rotating hips back) then relax the leg once it looses contact with the ground. There is a physics term called a 'moment arm' this refers to the amount of energy required to rotate an object. If the object (your knee, lower leg and foot) is more compact (i.e. not extended but flexed) it will require less energy to move backwards. Hence keeping your heel as close to your butt and rotating your knee forward back into high knee position will take much less energy, with this positioning. Secondly it also will create more elastic stored energy to propel you forward, with getting your knee higher, efficiently.

The key with all of these drills is to practice perfect technique, if you have perfect technique then gradually increase the movement speed. Start at 30-50% of your fastest movement speed, or slower if you still need to improve technique. Then add limb movement speed, (but not linear speed), and power output. Once you can perform the given drill at 85-95% of maximal output, with excellent technique you can advance or progress the drill. Generally speaking you can increase your intensity level by 10-15% per week. As I have always said to the runners/sprinters I have coached, if you can't do this technique perfectly standing still or at a slow walk then there is no way you can do it at 15 or 20mph, in fact you most likely will not achieve and maintain those speeds with out injury.

For coaches, look not only at the whole picture of movement but if the athlete is unbalanced, stiff, hips are breaking, or knees are rotating in. If so, go back to your musculoskeletal evaluation and look for the root cause and mobility/stability imbalance.

Remember some runners cannot do correct technique because their body does not allow them, address the underlying cause and it will clean up the dynamic stability problems and allow the advancement to increased intensity and complex movement patterns.

The best way to implement these drills into your training is:

Integrate drills into 2-3 training sessions per week, add one additional session each consecutive week till you are doing them most every day you run.

For each session- Start with an easy 1k warm-up, then move into drills. Remember something is always better than nothing so even 3 x 10m or 2 x 20m is better than not doing them at all. Once your technique is perfect then progress to the next level.

For Technique Videos go to http://www.e3sportsperformance.com

## Level 1

Repeat each drill 3 x 20m (meters).
**Key Points-** Knee-up, Toes Up (dorsi-flexed), impact ground under your hip, only increase movement speed and tempo when your technique is proficient, Movement over 20m should take 20-30 s (seconds).

Body Lean Drill

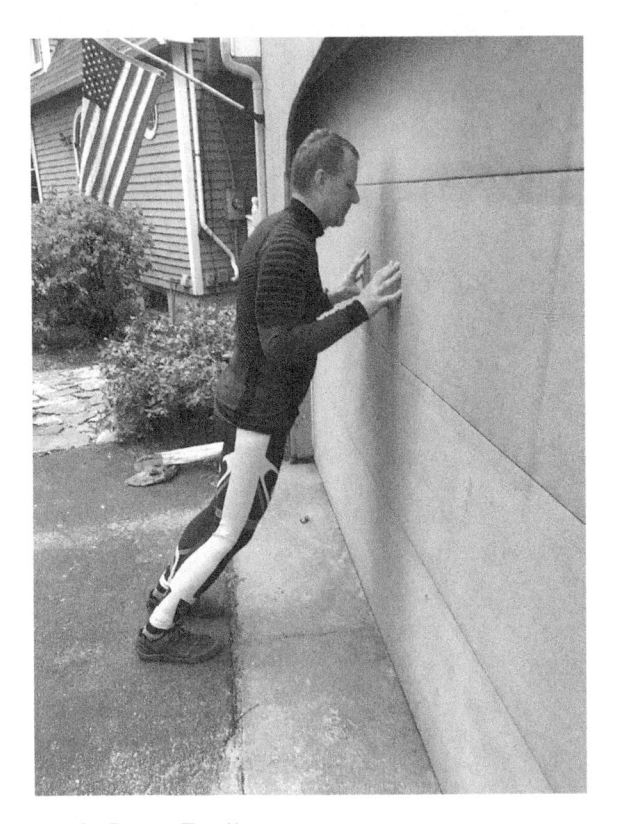

**Body Lean Drill-** Stand 2 ft from a wall, facing it, have hands at chest height. Squeeze butt cheeks, and lean forward from the ankle and have body 'fall' towards the wall. Repeat 10-15 times. To progress move outside to an 20% or greater incline, and fall forward take a short (6" step) and repeat alternating legs, when you feel comfortable link steps together to glide up hill with nice body lean.

Arm Swing Drill

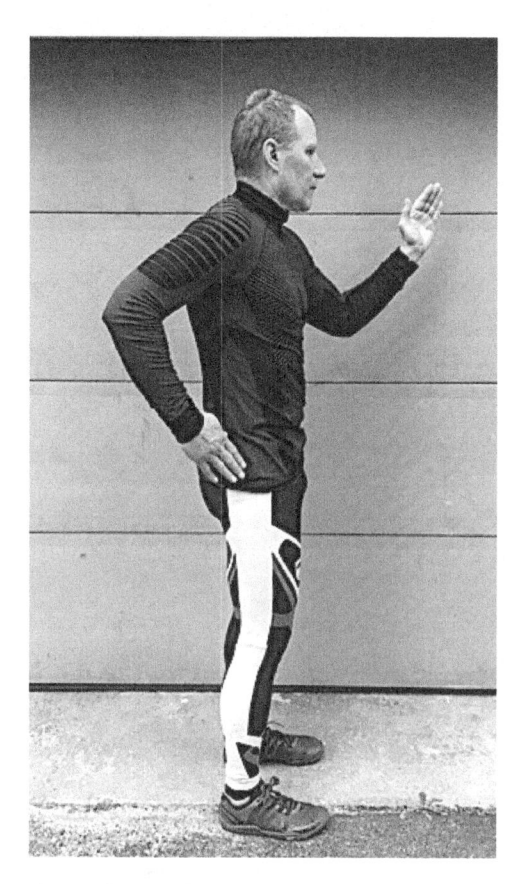

**Arm Swing Drill**- Standing or sitting on ground with legs extended, have- 90-100 degree bend in elbow, hand extended and relaxed, alternate swinging of arms first slow then gradually increasing speed (only if technique is perfect) rotation of arm comes from shoulder, fingertips at forward rotation should be level with eye/cheek, and butt cheek with backward rotation (cheek to cheek). Swing should be relaxed, yet snappy.

High Knee Walk

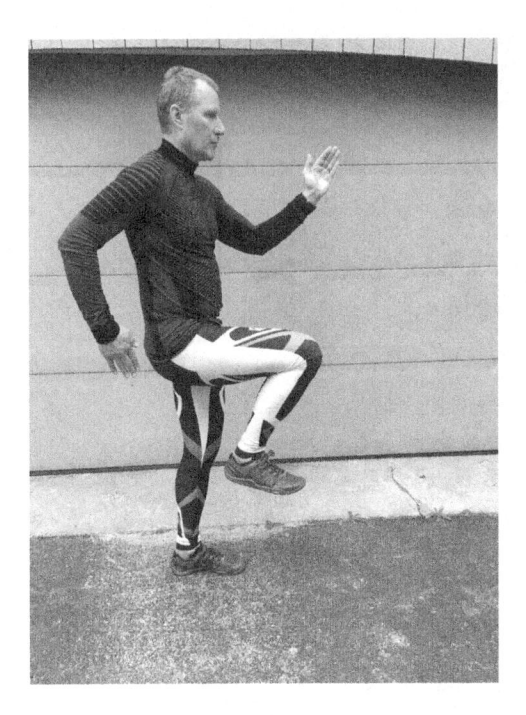

**High Knee Walk**-Goal of this drill is to develop perfect body position and technique with a full range of slow movements. Swing arm contralaterlaterally to knee swinging up. Bring thigh parallel to the ground, no higher, (as this creates vertical and backward lift forces). Make sure ankle is dorsiflexed, knee comes to 90 degrees, and arms have full swing. After hip flexion- let leg/foot relax and drop to ground, get the feeling of turning off the muscles and letting gravity have it fall. Have foot land right under hip next to weight bearing foot.

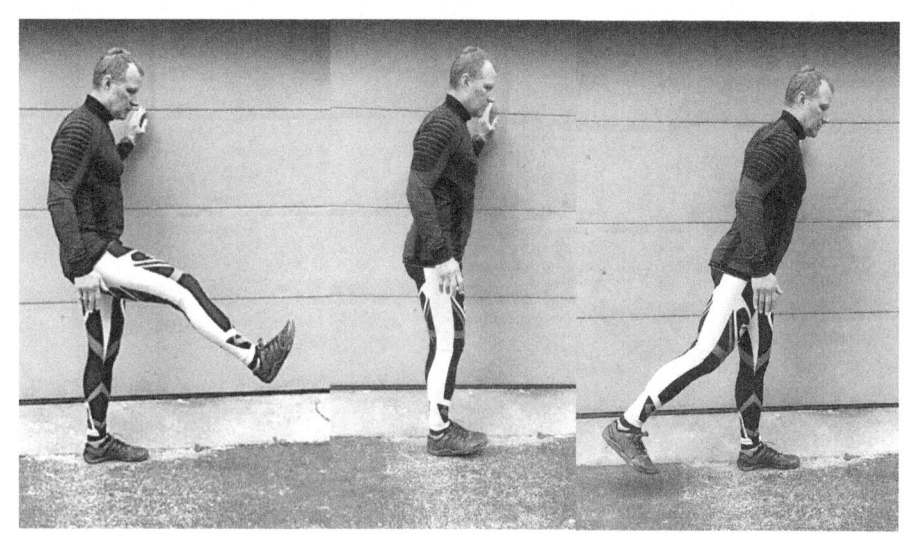

Clawing Drill Start     Contact under hip     Extension

**Clawing Drill** – Goal of this drill is to practice correct foot strike placement under your center of gravity. This is very important to master in order to decrease over-striding. Stand up have right hand touching wall or fence if needed, Have knee come up to 90 degrees, extend shin, dorsi-flex ankle (Keep toes up ) then sweep leg back. Make sure the foot contacts the ground only under the center of gravity or right next to the other foot. Keep ankle dorsiflexed throughout whole range of motion.

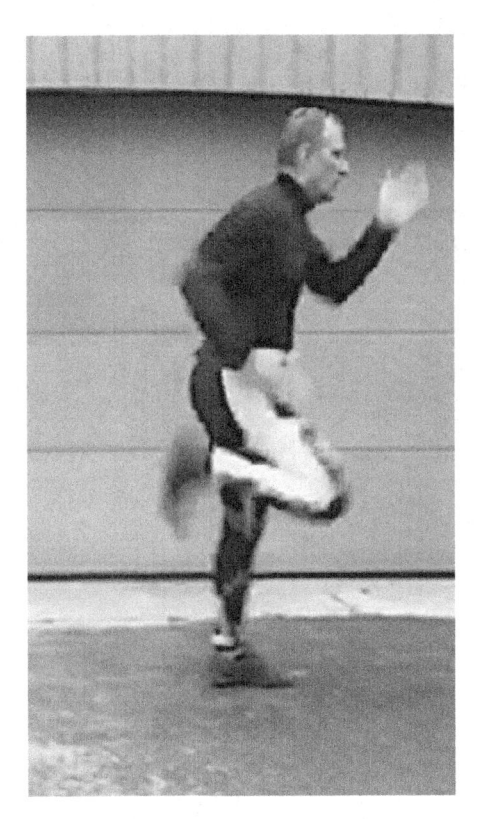

Butt Kick Drill

**Single leg Butt Kick**-Goal of this drill is to develop efficient recovery mechanics, and transfer free energy from power application phase to high knee phase. Move with a slow shuffle with for full arm drive pull/accelerate foot back to hit buttock with heel of foot. Focus on fast relaxed movement, coordinated with arm drive. Start with one leg, down 20m, then return with opposite leg. Should feel like you are scraping mud off bottom of shoe.

# Level 2

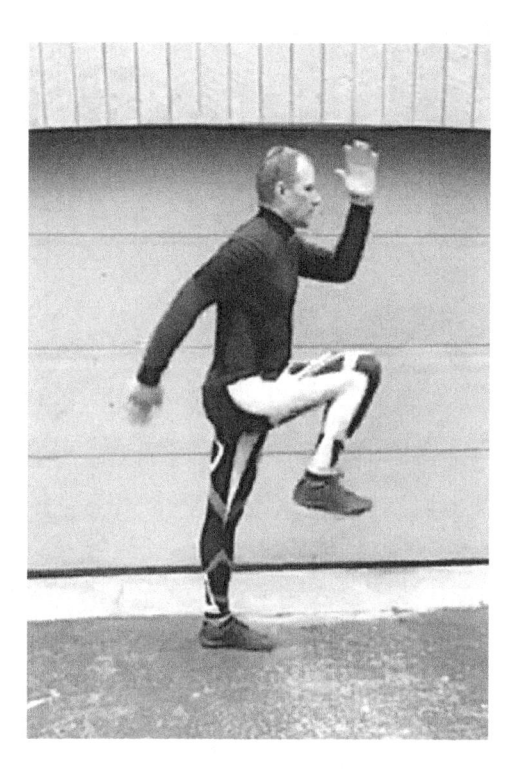

High Knee March

**High Knee March**- Increase High Knee Walking movement up to marching tempo, gradually increase speed as long as technique is excellent.

High Knee Skip

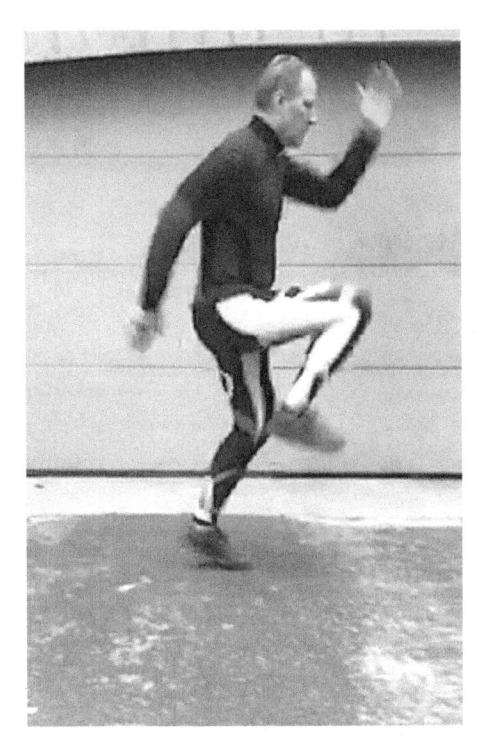

**High Knee Skip-** There are many different versions of this drill with different technical goals. This version the goal is to focus on a rapid acceleration of the knee up to fully flexed position, as this happens the runner should feel the weight bearing foot slide forward on the ground due to the accelerative forces of the knee drive. It is important to note that the weight bearing foot lift comes from the contralateral limb acceleration not a push off from the weight bearing foot.

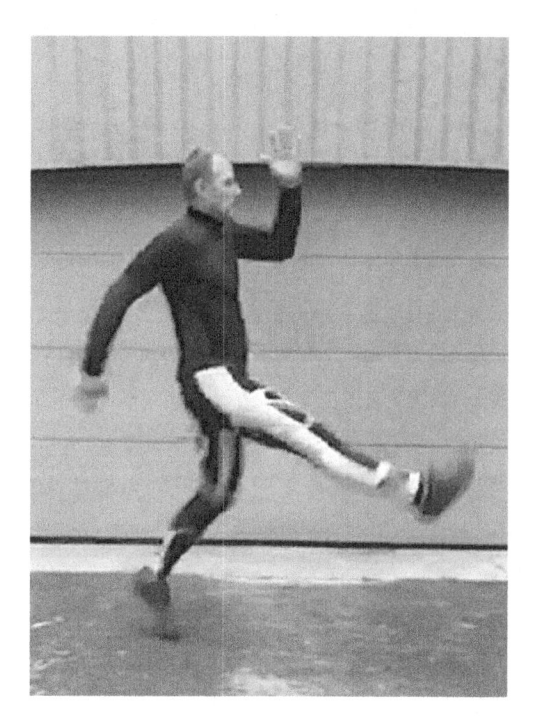

Scissor Drill

**Straight Leg Pull Through/Scissors-** Goal is to apply power right under the hip. Keep leg straight, lean back, while pulling through and contacting the ground under the hip with leg extended. Keep ankle dorsi-flexed. Start with 50% power output progress with consecutive sessions to apply more power with goal of having progressively longer stride lengths. Goal is to do as few strides as possible over 20m. (Note do not do this drill in spikes)

**Double Leg Butt kick-** Same drill as above, just alternating legs, (not in rapidly alternating movement) but shuffle-right leg-shuffle step left leg. Will take some practice to get a good rhythm.

# Level 3

**Alternating High Knees-** With same technique as high knee march drill, change tempo and rhythm to increase the movement frequency. Focus on excellent technique, increase limb speed only to the point of no technical decline (i.e. same knee height, keep ankle dorsi flexed, no reaching, foot impact under hip). As you move forward gradually increase high knee frequency, but make sure your linear velocity is slow. i.e. high knee movement speed increases, but the time to go 20m is still 5-8 seconds.

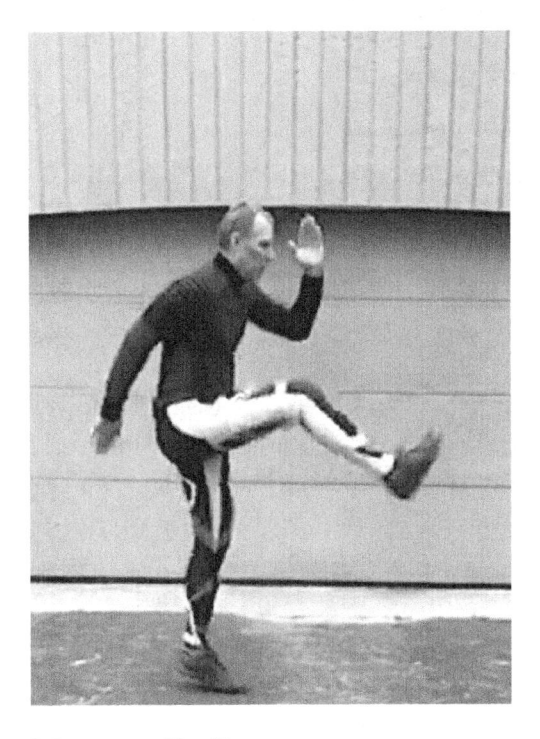

**Majorette Drill**

**Majorettes-** (Skip A/B) This is a combination of High knee and a Scissor drill. The proper rhythm and timing is essential. Initiate movement with a High Knee Skip then extend your leg and shin and sweep leg back quickly to contact the ground under your hip. Alternate legs.

**Double Leg Butt Kick with Increasing Acceleration**- Same movement as drill in Level-2 start with shuffling movement then as moving forward increase frequency by alternating legs and speeding up movement tempo.

## Injury Prevention and Footware

Another factor in injury prevention is running shoes. These days there seems to be as many different types and designs of running shoes and there are runners. It can be overwhelming if you are a new runner, or even seasoned runner just looking for good advice to be comfortable and injury free.
In Born to Run Christopher McDougall (2010) discussed how the incidence of running injuries increased with the development of modern running shoe design. He documented how many company's shoe designs were actually increasing injury risk. Research by Marti et al. (1984) found there was an increased injury rate with more expensive running shoes. Richards et al. (2009) found there was no evidence based research of shoe design supporting features such as heel cushioning and stability control systems. Research by Lieberman et al. (2010, 2015) found conventional running shoes actually increased impact forces by 2-3 times body weight and over-striding, when compared to barefoot running.

Less is better when it comes to running shoes and orthodics in preventing injury. The more we interfere with the natural movement of our feet and biomechanics the more we put our bodies at a risk of injury. Like wise a study by Ridge et al. (2015) found minimalist shoes increased running economy by 6.15%.

If you are biomechanically predisposed to injury- fix the underlying factors so you can run with the shoe that interferes with your natural mechanics the least. Adding more support, stability, and cushioning does not fix the underlying problem it only delays the inevitable running injury, which is why we see close to 75% of the runners injured each year. Start each season or any new activity with a good OS or FMS assessment, address your mobility stability issues and progress to running in a good minimalist shoe.

If you have been running for years in a high support or cushion shoe this transition needs to be done gradually. Anytime you buy new shoes you don't want to just put them on and run 20 miles! The change in your mechanics will induce some muscle soreness at the very least, or injury at the worst. Since any new shoe changes your mechanics for every stride, you need to phase the new shoe in over a couple weeks to prevent muscle soreness and injury. If you are used to a shoe with 1.5" of cushioning and are transitioning to a minimalist shoe then plan that transition over 6-12 months, as it will take this amount of time for your muscles to stretch and adapt to the changes. This transition will take time depending on the tightness of your posterior chain. After the transition you will be running faster and injury free in the long run. Net result make slow changes and your feet will be happy.

Minimalist shoes developed the reputation for increasing injury risk, this was related to; too fast a transition, especially in high mileage runners. The negative research studying injuries due to minimalist shoes was flawed due to poor controls and too rapid a change from conventional to minimalist shoes. Any rapid changes in mechanics with no reductions in training volume with the transition to new shoes will induce injury.

# 3

# The Building Blocks of Your Training Program

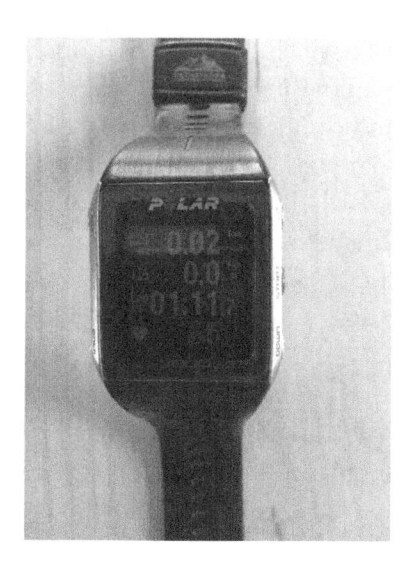

When I was in college my nordic coach, Cory Schwartz, used to say the key to training effectively for endurance sports is when you go slow, run real easy and when you go fast, run real fast, and don't do much of the in-between stuff. This is still dead-on advice to this day. Sounds simple enough but what does it really mean? If your training goal is to improve endurance then train at an easy level for 1.5 or more hours. Don't get into that intermediate zone, as little physiological adaption occurs there. We don't want to race *kind of* fast so why spend much time in the Level 3 zone? It does not develop the long-term capacity we need to race fast. Then for developing the ability for running fast, higher intensity training at Level 4 and above is what helps us develop the ability to run at a progressively higher pace for races.

To monitor and quantify our training load we need to utilize some key tools. At the very least you need a basic heart rate monitor that uses a chest strap to get an accurate heart rate measurement. Being a scientist at heart, I always opt for more data; so if you can, spring for a heart rate monitor (HRM) that has GPS, because then you can easily tag your performance metrics to multiple data points. Knowing that you kept your heart rate within Level 1 is important, but if in five weeks you are running at the same heart rate on the same terrain/conditions and your average speed is 5% faster, then you have solid evidence that your training program is working. The other nice feature of HRMs is the ability to upload the data into your training log. This allows you to have a good system of organization of your training data and ability to effectively track your performance gains.

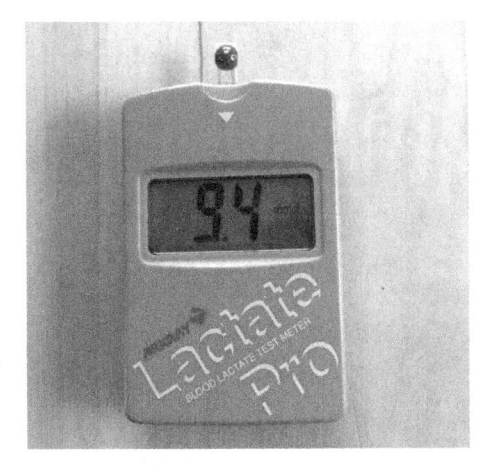

The second tool is a portable lactate analyzer. I recommend this if you are really spending a lot of time training and want the gold standard of measuring performance changes.

## Endurance Training

Endurance training is the foundation of aerobic exercise. It develops our cardiovascular system and aerobic enzymatic base so that we can maintain a high workload aerobically. Physiologists used to think that all these adaptations occurred only by training high volumes of long, slow distance in Level 1 and Level 2, however, over the years we have learned that some of these adaptations occur at higher intensities of exercise as well. Easy training hours develop our aerobic base. The most important are improvements in our cardiovascular system, improved aerobic metabolism, and development of aerobic enzymes. We develop better blood circulation to our muscles with increased capillaries, increased mitochondrial density, and increased aerobic enzymes/biochemical changes. With continuous repetition we develop technical efficiency. These long hours are also the ideal time to develop efficient technique. Our bodies learn how to run relaxed and efficiently when we are fatigued, which is a significant factor to racing fast as well.

If you are training for longer races (marathon or ultra) we need to develop the capacity to run these distances efficiently, which can happen only by putting in longer hours to develop and improve our aerobic muscular capacity.

## Intensity Training

Intensity training helps us develop the ability to maintain a high race pace for a longer period of time. There is a spectrum of intensity training from Level 3 (sub-lactate to lactate threshold) to Level 8 (sprint training). Each level develops a specific range of physiological capacity; there are crossover adaptations to higher and lower intensity levels of fitness. As the season progresses you will spend more time doing your intensity training at race pace or above. This does not mean you will not train these abilities earlier in the season. This area is a bit of where the coaching art can take over. For example, for every athlete there will be a unique combination of intensity training that is optimal just for them. Much of this can be determined by testing. Sometimes faster adaptations can occur with higher intensity levels, but this is very individual-specific determined by one's physiological base, physiological makeup, and regenerative capacity. There is some trial and error, hence the importance of having a training log so you can look back and see what type of training gave you a really big bang in performance.

After twenty years of coaching I have found that many endurance athletes can benefit a great deal from higher intensity speed work. There are strong neuromuscular adaptations from higher intensity and sprint work that can generalize over to improved motor efficiency. It is important to have an excellent strength and power base before integrating this type, to be injury resistant. Even in the early season I will integrate high intensity workouts for some of the microcycles. In some athletes this can stimulate a supercompensation. If so then consider increasing the frequency of these training sessions throughout the year.

## Tempo, Interval Training, and Speed Training: What to Use and When

### Interval Training

### Tempo Training Level 3

As I discussed earlier, I don't recommend having tons of hours of training in this zone, mainly because we develop little physiological capability here. For beginner/developing athletes that have not had much structured training, tempo is a good way to transition into more structured, higher intensity interval training. This training zone develops your capacity just below your lactate threshold. If you find that in your lactate testing you jumped up in a few heart beats from your aerobic zones right into 4 mmol of lactate, you could benefit from training in this zone. It is also a way to develop efficiency just below race pace. This can also be applied early season to do some fun and natural interval-type workouts. The goal here is to have efficient technique at this higher workload. This is a good time to emphasize snappy technique but still maintain fluid, economical movements. The rest interval between repetitions is two minutes. With easy active rest you recover faster, when your heart rate drops to 120, you can start your next repeat.

## Interval Training Level 4 and Level 5

The goal of these training sessions is to stimulate an adaptation of efficiency and work capacity at lactate threshold. The adaptations we are trying to stimulate here is efficiency in a high state of lacticity, and increased lactate buffering capacity. When we look at lactate curves we are trying to create a rightward shift where at the same heart rate you produce less lactate (because your body has adapted and improved its buffering capacity). Longer interval times are designed to train just at or above your LT; shorter interval times are focused on stimulating higher tolerances (i.e., above race pace) of lactate.

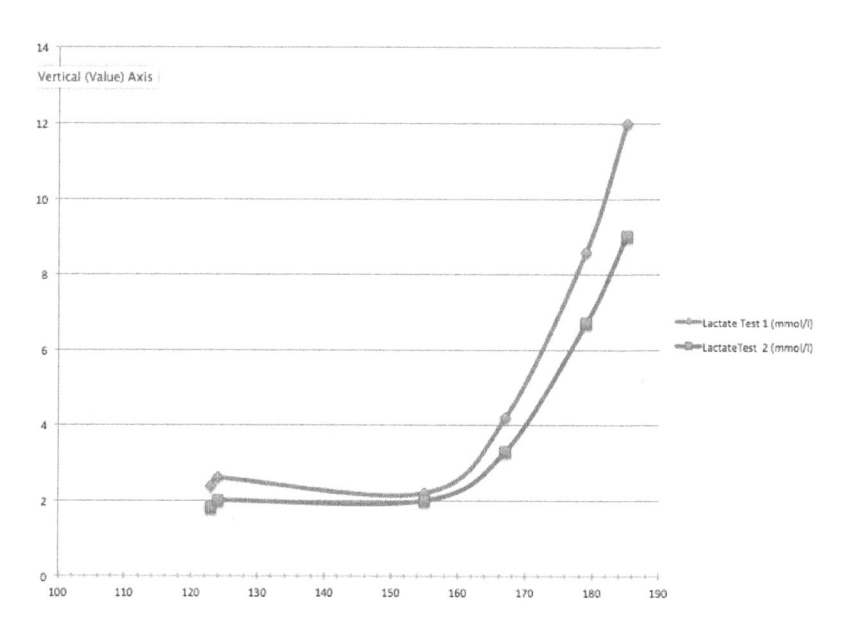

*Graph 1: Changes in lactate with interval training*

Rightward shift in test 2 after three months of interval training represents increased lactate tolerance for same heart rate. For performance this runner started at a lactate level of 4.2 mmol at a 5:23 mile pace, which changed to 3.3 mmol at a 5:23 mile pace.

**Key Points for Interval Training**

- For interval repeats use the same start point for each circuit/loop. The goal is to go longer/faster with each consecutive interval (remember your HRM data?) with the goal to run the longest with your last repeat. This allows you to have a tangible performance goal. It also allows you to see how technical changes impact your running efficiency.

- After your last repeat you should always feel like you could do two more repeats at the same speed and HR. You should never feel totally wiped out after an interval workout, for example.

- To increase intensity, change only one variable at a time (time of interval, number of repeats, recovery time). Decrease increased difficulty of terrain (increased vertical climb per interval). This so you can determine what gave you the biggest bang for your training.

- To initially boost intensity, increase the number of repeats (but do not exceed 20-25 minutes total time interval time unless you are an elite athlete).

- Increase time under stress by increasing your interval time: 4:00 to 4:30, 5:00 to 5:30, etc.

- Start with a good warm-up, 7 to 10 minutes in L1-2, then do 3 to 5 sprints to increase your heart rate

When and how do you progress your intervals? When you have adapted to the present load and you are going 5% or greater distance over the same time, course, and HR that you started at initially.

What you do to progress your intervals depends upon your goals and fitness profile. If your goal is to increase your lactate buffering capacity, first assess the progress of your adaptation with some lactate spot testing at your LT. If your capacity has increased you can increase the intensity of your interval repeats to a higher HR, extend the time of the interval, or decrease your rest interval from three minutes to two and a half minutes, then two minutes, or increase difficulty/incline of terrain.

How long is too long for intervals at the L5 intensity level? Research by Larsen and Jenkins (2002) and (Helgerud,, et. al, 2007) found that for non-elite athletes four minutes is the magic number, but more advanced and higher trained athletes can extend this time up to seven minutes. Most athletes do not have the capacity to maintain a high pace beyond seven minutes, hence there is no value to exceeding this.

## Keeping the Workouts Fun

- Vary the location and terrain of your intervalsSwitch the mode up by mixing with hiking, cycling, As you get closer to the competitive season, get more specificTrain with a club or friends

## Frequent Mistakes with Intervals

- Going too hard too soon. This is a transition into consistently having 2–3 intensity workouts a week. Like all of your training, if implemented correctly it will be enjoyable.

- Train in the right zone. If your HR is too high then you are not achieving the goal of this training. You also run the risk of doing muscle damage if you are at too high of a lactate level.

- Don't try to hit that target zone in the first 30 seconds. You will dump too much lactate into your system and the rest of your workout will be compromised. The first 1.5–2 minutes of the interval, you are building into your HR target zone.
- Take the recommended rest interval until you adapt to the intensity load.

## Where to Start?

As we discussed earlier, you should have a basic road map in hand from your baseline physiological evaluation. A good coach would be able to give you advice on where to focus your efforts for intensity training. If resources or access to an experienced coach are not an option, below are some guidelines to help you in making your decision.

If you are new to interval training or have not done much intensity training, your best bet is to start out with a transition phase into intervals. This would start with 2–3 weeks of tempo training, 2 sessions for the first week then 2-3 sessions the following week. Start with the minimum volume of 6–8 minutes with 2 minutes active rest between each repeat, then increase the length of the repeat (i.e., go from 8–10 minutes for each repeat). Your third week you can add in one session of interval training 3 x 3 minutes at a higher intensity with 3 minutes of rest.

Advanced athletes with a strong training base could start with L4 interval sessions. For example, 4 x 3.5 mins in L4 with 3 minutes of active rest.

## Sample Interval Sessions

*Early season or preparatory phase*

3x3 mins: Level 4–5, active rest for 3 minutes

3x4 mins: Level 4–5, active rest for 4 minutes

*Preseason or after 2–3 months of structured intensity training*

4x4 mins: Level 5, rest 3–4 minutes (or until HR has dropped to 120)

4x5 mins: Level 5, rest 3–4 minutes (or until HR has dropped to 120)

## Intensity Blocks

Intensity blocks are an advanced form of training where an athlete does multiple consecutive days of interval training in L4–5. For well-trained athletes this can stimulate a rapid adaptation to increase stroke volume and lactate tolerance to increase VO2 max by 5% over a 7–10 day period in elite athletes (Aalberg, 2002).

The key to the successful implementation of this training system is not exceeding lactate levels of 4–10 mmols, for each repeat. Otherwise early in the sessions you will not be able to maintain the same high-level work output. The mode of training must be systematically changed to not over-fatigue one muscle group. You must have one rest day after every 2–3 intensity sessions.

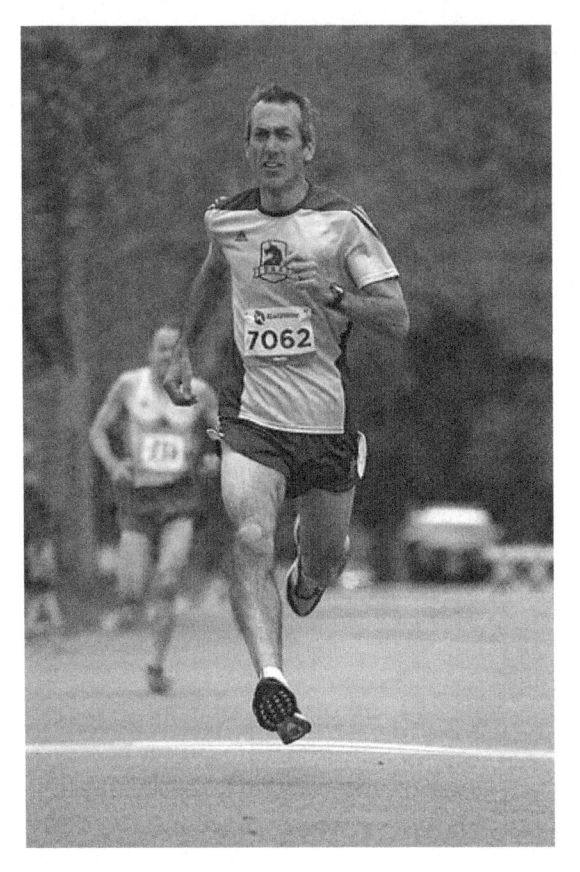

*Peter Hammer 2016 Great Bear Run* **(Courtesy of Peter Hammer)**

*Intensity Block Example (Karlsen and Aalberg, 2004)*

**Day 1:** 4 x 3:00 minutes at HR 85 – 90% of MHR (3 minutes at HR 60% in between bursts) (3 mins recovery between repetitions)
**Day 2:** 3 x 3:30 minutes at HR 90% of MHR (3:30 mins recovery between repetitions)
**Day 3:** Recovery (rest or 30 minutes easy run, bike, row, or hike)
**Day 4:** 4 x 3:00 minutes at HR 90% of MHR (3 mins recovery between repetitions)
**Day 5:** 4 x 3:30 minutes at HR 85 - 90% of MHR (3:30 mins recovery between repetitions)

**Day 6:** Recovery (rest or 30 minutes easy run, bike, row, or hike)
**Day 7:** Recovery (rest or 30 minutes easy run, bike, row, or hike)
**Day 8:** 4 x 3:30 minutes at HR 90% of MHR (3:30 mins recovery between repetitions)
**Day 9:** 3 x 4:00 minutes at HR 85 – 90% of MHR (4 mins recovery between repetitions)
**Day 10:** 2 x 5 minutes at HR 85 – 90% of MHR (5 mins recovery between repetitions)

**Pros:** Intensity blocks when properly implemented can stimulate a rapid adaptation and increase in fitness.

**Cons:** If the runner goes too hard, especially in the early interval repetitions or sessions, they can dump too much lactate into their muscles and not only do muscle damage, but if they continue to repeat high intensity efforts, can end up having a marked long term decrease in performance.

# Strength Training

Strength and power training are two distinct yet interdependent elements of physiological development. Strength is the foundation of power and should be the first step in the development of a sound base from which the athlete can progress their training into more advanced exercises. The most important benefit of strength and power training is the development of increased force output of the muscles.

For master-level runners, strength training is an underutilized tool for development, especially given the effects of aging. In addition, there are hormonal adaptations, which will benefit regeneration and recovery as well.

For all runners, especially developing and masters runners the most important aspect of strength development is core strength. For years, as coaches and physiologists, we have been focused on more speed, power, strength, and endurance. However, all this work is not optimized if we don't have the fundamental ability to generate power, transfer it effectively between joints then into the ground, and have optimal mobility to use the full length of all of our muscle fibers effectively.

Reflexive core strength is the foundation of efficient movement patterns. Hip stabilization and coordinating segmented movements between the upper and lower body is primarily mediated/controlled by our deep pelvic floor and transverse abdominal muscles. The key is to keep the core exercises dynamic and reflexive (it is reflexes that drive the optimal functioning of the deep reflexive core). Good running technique does not consist of doing static planking for five minutes. The exercise needs to be dynamic, hence you need to lift an arm, leg, or both (with proper body alignment) to keep the plank reflexive. It is important to do perfect technique. It is far more effective to do perfect technique for three seconds versus poor technique for 30 seconds (this just keeps reinforcing the dysfunctional muscle firing pattern!).

Once the runner has a well developed foundation of core strength and mobility they can progress to a program that blends more advanced reflexive core strength exercises with conventional strength exercises. Conventional strength training is necessary to strengthen the muscles, tendons and ligaments. This phase is critical in being injury resistant prior to progressing to power and speed training.

For Core and Strength Training Videos go to http://www.e3sportsperformance.com

**Core Strength Exercises**
3 Sets 8-12 Repetitions

Dead Bug
Super-Dog

Incline Plank
Glute-Pull
Cook Hip-Lift
Loaded Crawls

**Strength Exercises-**
3 Sets 10-12 Repetitions

-Romanian (single-leg) dead lifts
-Step ups
-Standing calf raises
-Kettle-bell swings
-Pull-ups
-1/2 Turkish Getups
Dips

For foundational strength the best way to start is with a base phase of 3 sets 10-12 repetitions to failure. After eight weeks of this phase the runner can progress to a power phase and some strength-power training complexes. This will transfer the general strength developed into functional power output increases. For this phase repetitions will be decreased to 4-6 reps, continuing with 3 sets, with the last repetition to failure (but with perfect technique). Many endurance athletes are concerned with gaining muscle mass and having a decrease in endurance performance. This is not the case. Since the dominant muscle fiber type and stimulation pattern in endurance athletes is endurance based they will have little increase in muscle mass. Any gains in muscle mass will increase running efficiency, hence there is a net gain in performance.

## Power Training

Power training through the application of plyometrics and strength power complex exercises is the most effective way to transfer strength gains to functional, specific running performance improvement. Prior to starting any power exercises it is important to have a solid strength base of at least six months. This is important to be injury resistant with more dynamic exercises. The tendons, especially at the myotendinous junction, need time to be strengthened to manage the forces of explosive power training. Many athletes tend to advance power exercises too rapidly which will lead to injury. It is critical to have a coach monitor the application and technique of these exercises to prevent injury. It is important that the neuromuscular and musculoskeletal system can adapt to the load, hence you want to start off slow. The important part is that you are able to manage these forces with good body position. The most crucial indicator of this is if your heels are hitting the ground when you are landing. If they are and you cannot stay on the balls of your feet then you will need to continue with strength development exercises longer.

## How to Start and Progress

Given the above operating principles, power training can be initiated and progressed in the following manner-

### Level 1
-Start with 1–2 sets of 5–10 jumps) with the most basic movements such as double leg hops (forward/backward, side to side). Rest 2 minutes between each set.
Exercises can be done just after warm-up just before you strength train.

-Progress by increasing your training volume first from 1-2 sets to 3 then 4 sets

### Level 2
-After 3-4 weeks increase intensity by doing 1-2 sets of single leg hops. Start with 2 sets then increase in consecutive weeks.

Make sure heel is not hitting the ground, then increase volume again after 2-3 weeks.

## Level 3
This progression is to increase intensity again by increasing jump height by doing box jumps. Start with a 6" box doing double leg hops, then progress to single leg hops as above. Start with 2 sets then increase in consecutive weeks. Make sure heel is not hitting the ground, then increase volume again after 2-3 weeks.

## Level 4
Increase box height by 6" to 12 ", then start back with double leg hops. The best we to do this transition is have half of your jumps still on a 6" box then the other half double leg on a 12" box.

Start with 2 sets then increase in consecutive weeks. Make sure heel is not hitting the ground, then increase volume again after 2-3 weeks.

## **KEY POINTS**

-Focus on precision and speed of movement

-Intensity of effort should be 95-100% (as the goal is to fire as much fast twitch muscle as possible

-Increase volume first, but only do a 10-15% increase per week to a maximum of 40-50 contacts per leg.

-Make sure your heel is not hitting the ground if it is then STOP, at this point the amortization phase is too long and you are not developing power, only strength.

-Once you have mastered 12" box jumps you can progress to more advanced power training exercises such as bounding

## Speed Training

Speed training in level 6-8 is a very effective method for improving neuromuscular efficiency, which generalizes over to improved running velocity at race pace. What I have found is there are strong responders and minimal responders to this stimulus. Much has to do with the individual physiological makeup and training base.

There are many different methods of applying speed training. We will discuss the basics in this section, then advanced methods in the second book.

**Prerequisites for Speed Training-** It is critical that before you start any speed training exercises that you have developed your strength, power, and technique foundation. Without this foundation you will develop an injury as you are putting a much higher level of stress on your musculoskeletal system.

The best training phase to implement speed training for beginner runners is in the pre-competition and competition phases of training. More advanced runners should be doing some level of speed training year round, with specifically focused macrocycles interspersed throughout the year then especially in the pre-competition and competition phases.

Speed Workout Structure –. Remember the goal is to finish the workout fatigued but not to the point that you could not run another 5k easy. With speed workouts the goal is not training volume but quality, hence each workout should not exceed 1200-1500 meters of high intensity running. After a short transition phase of 1-2 weeks, test your times for 30m, 60m, 100m, 200, and 400m to determine a baseline reference point for your training time percentages.

Start each speed workout with an Easy 1500m warm-up run

-Dynamic Mobility
-Stride Development Drills

5x 30m ( 85-90%)
5 x 60m (85-90%)

4x100m ( 85%)
2x200m (85%)

1000-1500m Warm down

The best way to progress your speed workouts is to start by increasing the intensity of your shorter distances from 90% to 95%, then 98 and 100%. Next stage would be to add in a power complex where bounding exercises are added in judiciously. The next stage would be to increase longer distance intensity to 90, 95, then 100%, after that you could gradually increase the distances (100m to 120m, 200m to 250 then 300m).

**Key Points**

- Intensity levels are based upon value of your maximal effort for that specific distance (30m, 60m 100m, 200m, 400m)
- Don't start speed work until your technique is well developed and you have a good strength and power base. You will risk injury as well as reinforce bad motor programs with more force.
- Do speed workouts in spikes (with a very slow transition to using these, i.e. increase volume in spikes by 100m per workout)
- Start in terrain that is slightly uphill so you can initially focus on power output, then progress to track where you can work on peak velocity.

- Pay close attention to your technical efficiency. Only go a distance that you can run well. Start with 5- to 10-second buildup sprints, then increase time up to 60 seconds and longer. Start with buildup sprints where you gradually accelerate to top speed with a focus on relaxed, snappy, and efficient technique.

- Focus on relaxed technique. Oftentimes, with exerting a high intensity effort we tighten up, lose body position, and then end up with fast and inefficient movements (this is where having a speed measurement is helpful).

- Utilize a GPS-based HRM so you can see velocity/heart rate relationship.

- For speed work, rest intervals range from 1:4–1:25 depending on the sprint time individual recovery time and intensity level.

- Increase number of repetitions or sprint time when you can sustain a maximal velocity for your existing workout load. Make sure with the new workload there is a slowing of your maximal velocity. Remember: quality over quantity.

- Over 40-60 seconds per repeat of sprinting will not develop your peak velocity. At this point you are training a different energy system (speed endurance) and it is not speed work, but a workout focused on peak lactate buffering capacity.

Additional and more advanced strength, power, and speed training concepts will be presented in the companion book, as these topics require much more in-depth coverage in order to be implemented effectively and safely.

## Multi-Dimensional Periodization for Running

The goal of multi-dimensional periodization is to have all of the training elements work together synergistically, and bridge adaptations from general to specific fitness. We are all familiar with distance training, tempo, speed—but how do they all fit together? How do they complement one another and help one become a faster runner?

In a given microcycle and workout it is important that all of the training activities work together. We know from physiological research that when certain elements are combined together in one workout, or in sequence, they will stimulate a stronger adaptation; the opposite is true as well. Much of this is driven by principles of neuromuscular-based training. For example, you would not want to do an interval or power workout right after a long endurance run since the fatigue level of the muscles would not allow a high level work output. On the other hand, when you combine power with speed (a speed-power complex), then the neuromuscular system is activated to a higher level and there is an adaptation to increased speed. Similarly with strength and power.

The ideal training combinations are:

- Power/Interval session: For example, doing 3 x 30m of bounding prior to a running interval workout will stimulate an increased force output of the running stride.
- Power/Speed: Bounding combined with speed work.
- Strength/Power: Strength exercises complexed with power exercises. An example is doing pull-ups followed by med-ball throw-downs.
- Speed/Strength/Power- this is an advanced training complex that combines all three components into a speed workout

*General principles*

1) To improve an element of running, you should focus on developing only two elements in a given microcycle. Reason

being is that the body can only adapt adequately to two stress loads at a given time.

2) Have element sequences complement each other. For example, don't do a lot of plyometrics prior to technique because the body will be too fatigued to perform good technique. Instead, apply technique early in the workout, then do the plyometrics.

3) Combine similar training elements, technique/endurance, speed/power, strength/power.

## Training Plan Examples

### Beginner Runner

*Prepatory Phase*

Monday: Off

Tuesday: Stride development drills then L1-2 Easy run 20-30 mins, finish with core strength

Wednesday: Running natural intervals 4 x 3 minutes, 3 minutes rest, finish with general strength

Thursday: L1–2 Run or Hike 30-40min

Friday: Off or Stride development drills then 20-min L2 run

Saturday: L4–5 Hill Running or natural intervals 3 x 3 minutes, 3 min rest, finish with core and general strength

Sunday: L1 hike 1.5–3+ hours

**Intermediate to Advanced Runner**
*Prepatory Phase*

Monday: Off

Tuesday: Stride development drills then, Running intervals 4 x 3 min, 2–3 min rest, finish with core strength

Wednesday: Stride development drills then, Running intervals 4 x 4 minutes, 2–3 minutes rest, finish with general strength

Thursday: L1–2 run 60 min, include Stride development drills

Friday: Off or 30-min L2 run

Saturday: L4–5 Stride development drills then, Running intervals on Hills 4 x 4 minutes, 2–3 min rest, finish with core and general strength

Sunday: L1 hike 2–3+ hours


**Beginner Runner**
*PreCompetition Competition*

Monday: Off or easy strength workout

Tuesday: Stride development drills then Speed training workout if you have the training base, if not then do L4 Interval workout 3 x 3-4mins with 3-4 mins recovery. Finish with core strength and 1-2 strength exercises for hamstrings and upper body.

Wednesday: Lower-body power training, then L1-2 Run with focus on good stride tempo (85-90 strides per minute)

Thursday: Stride development drills then, L1 Run 40-60 minutes

Friday: Lower-body power training, then L4 Hill Running repeats 4 x 3-4 minutes with 3-4 minutes rest

Saturday: L1 hike 2–3+ hours

Sunday: Stride development drills then L2 Run with technique focus 30 mins, Finish with core strength and 1-2 strength exercises for hamstrings and upper body. 30 mins

**Intermediate to Advanced Runner**
*PreCompetition*

Monday: Off

Tuesday: Stride development drills then Speed training workout, followed by max strength workout
Wednesday: Stride development drills then, L1-L2 Run 60-80 minutes

Thursday: L4-5 Running Intervals, 4 x 4-5 minutes with 2 minutes rest, finish with 2-3 max strength exercises

Friday: Lower-body power training, then L3 Hill Running repeats 4 x 4 minutes with 2-3 minutes rest, finish with core strength

Saturday: L1 hike 2–3+ hours

Sunday: Stride development drills then L2 Run with technique focus 30-60 mins, core strength 30 mins

Sometimes, despite our best plans and intentions, our days can go sideways and our training plans are thrown off. With bailout workouts something is always better than nothing. For an interval day one quick option is a 10-minute high-intensity workout. Start with a 5-minute warm-up, then transition into 2 x 4-minute intervals or 1 x 8–10 minutes. Finish with a 5-minute warm-down.

If you missed a long endurance workout and you have an intensity day the next day, 10–15 minutes of core strength and mobility will be a great quick way to keep building your base while keeping you fresh for the next workout.

# 4

# Junior-Level Runner Development

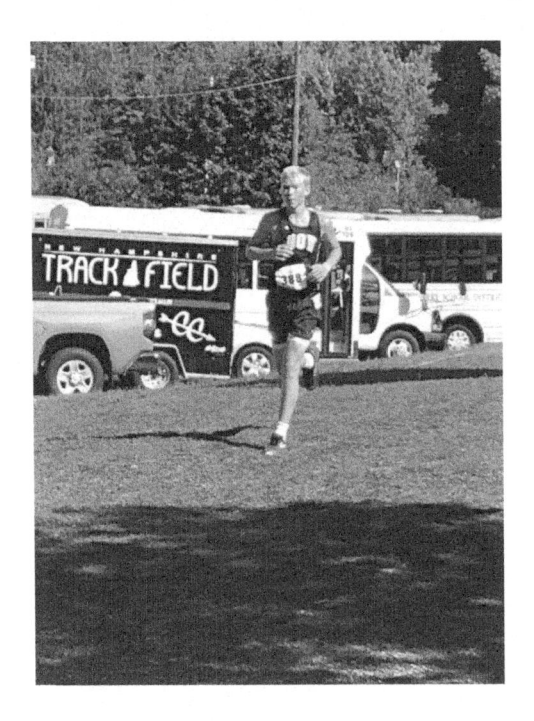

Junior-level runners are still developing their physiological base so they need a different developmental approach than master-level runners. For starters pre-pubertal runners do not have the fundamental enzymatic capability to buffer lactate at higher levels; these enzymes develop during puberty, hence adaptations to high intensity interval training are minimal. (Viru et al., 1999) The primary developmental goals are focused on the development of endurance, strength, power, and technique. Youth athletes are unique in their age-sensitive developmental training adaptations, where at different ages, they are much more receptive to different types of training stimuli. For example, you get a big bang of development if you emphasize a given training element at a certain age range. This is very important when we look at gender. Age-sensitive development is an area that continues to remain untapped in the developmental process of many junior-level runners. It is rarely utilized in the development of junior-level athletes in the US and when employed, can yield exceptional long-term performance gains.

## Age-Sensitive Development of Youth

"Training is most effective when it stimulates maturing abilities rather than those already matured"(Drabik, 1989).

Teaching youth runners skills and running movement patterns can be optimized with the application of some basic motor learning principles. Improving their overall athletic development can also be optimized if we integrate the principles of age-sensitive development. Age-sensitive development refers to periods of time in a youth's life where they are much more receptive to developing certain fundamental neuromuscular skills (balance, timing, rhythm, coordination, and speed of movement). If the child is stimulated with a given element in this receptive time they will develop this skill much more rapidly. When this is done there are very rapid biomotor and physiological adaptations of children when stimulated/trained at highly receptive age ranges. For example, training limb speed at the ages of 7–10 over 8–12 months will have the same gains as several years of training at the age of 19.

The largest amount of neuromuscular development in youth occurs between the ages of 3–16 and is in the nervous system. This is the optimal period for balance, rhythm, motor engram, speed, and power development. These are known as the child's "Golden Years." Since the nervous system controls all of the functioning of our muscles, we have a great deal to benefit from this.

Why would we train youth in this manner versus conventional means? The major reason for application of these principles is it will lead to much greater advancement and development of foundation abilities in youth athletes. **When we train athletes in more receptive periods we make gains in months that would normally take years at a different age.**

It will optimize:

- Neuromuscular development
- Physiological development
- Strength development
- Injury prevention
- Rapid development of foundation abilities of youth
- Increased neuromuscular plasticity

An increased focus on the neuromuscular development of youth athletes will improve the foundation skills of:

- Balance
- Rhythm
- Coordination
- Agility
- Speed

# History

Throughout the 1960s and 1970s a great deal of empirical research was conducted in Eastern Bloc countries on the development of youth athletes. Data was extensively gathered on the efficacy of different methods of training. Through the application of different coaching/training methods of youth athletes over many years, much was learned about the neuromuscular physiology of youth athletes. New theories were developed, tested, and refined. This led to major advancements in training theory and methodology for youth. Much of this research could not be duplicated present day due to regulations of research on human subjects.

# Skill Development and Motor Learning

Development of a motor skill is dependent upon several variables:

1) The complexity of the skill

2) One's base level of learning

3) The level of motor development

For a runner to learn a complex skill it takes about two years. Perfection takes an infinite amount of time. Elite runners require 10,000 hours of development. Simple skills take about 2–3 months to learn.

"The acquisition of a skill does not occur at once, but rather through three phases: During the first phase, on the basis of a poor neuromuscular coordination, useless movements occur. A dispersion of nervous impulses beyond the normal path of conduction stimulates supplementary muscles. The coach should not misjudge the lack of neuromuscular coordination as insufficient talent potential, but rather as a physiological reality. 2-The phase of tensed movements; and 3- The phase of establishing a motor skill through an adequate coordination of the nervous processes. Thus, the skill or the dynamic stereotype is formed" (Krestovnikov, 1951 in Bompa, 1990).

The fourth level of skill development is the mastery of the skill which is "characterized by performing fine movements with high efficiency as well as the ability to adapt the skill to eventual environment changes" (Bompa, 1990). Learning of the skill takes a great deal of time and practice (i.e., thousands of repetitions). This is what takes the skill from a cerebral level (thinking about the technique as you do it) to the cerebellar level (having the motion become automatic or reflexive).

It is important for the coach to know how to manipulate the neural load for skill development. Since running has such a large technical component, manipulating the proprioceptive load variables is a good means of teaching/improving technique, thus accelerating the learning process. One way to improve one's balance is to increase the proprioceptive load by removing one of the elements of balance. One's balance consists of neuromuscular feedback, our visual field, and vestibular motor feedback. Removing one of those factors increases the load on the other variables. Doing balance drills with your eyes closed will create a higher load on the other senses. Another means of training this is to change the feedback characteristics of the environment, as the environment is constantly changing. An example of this would be to do balance drills on the sand, snow, or in bare feet (but not in the snow!). Last but not least you can try to force the athlete out of balance through the tossing of a ball, or pulling on the torso or limb with a TheraBand. Contrasting drills and proprioceptive loads can improve the speed of balance and skill acquisition.

## Motor Skill/Technique Development

The Golden Years of neuromuscular development are from 6–13 years of age. This is the optimal period for motor engram development and patterning of motor skills. This is not to say that at later ages this does not happen, but the acquisition of motor skill will just take longer at older ages.

## Sensitive Periods of Coordination Training

- Balance: 10–11 males, 9–10 females
- Movement adequacy: 8–13 both sexes
- Kinesthetic differentiation (ability to correctly estimate differences in form, timing, distance, and strength modulation): 6–7, then 10–11
- Reaction time: 8–10
- Rhythmic motion: 9–10 males, 7–9 females
- Spatial orientation: 12–14
- Synchronization of movements in time: 6–8

| Age<br>F-Female<br>M-Male | 6-8 | | 8-9 | | 9-10 | | 10-11 | | 11-12 | | 12-13 | | 13-14 | | 14-15 | | 15-16 | | 16-17 | |
|---|---|---|---|---|---|---|---|---|---|---|---|---|---|---|---|---|---|---|---|---|
| | F | M | F | M | F | M | F | M | F | M | F | M | F | M | F | M | F | M | F | M |
| Balance | | | | | H | | | H | | | FM | | FM | | FM | | FM | | FM | |
| Rhythm | H | | H | | | | H | | H | | | | | | | | | | | |
| Movement Adequecy | | | | | | | H | | H | | H | | H | | H | | | | | |
| Synchronization of Movements in Time | H | H | | | | | | | | | | | | | | | | | | |
| Coordination | | | | | H | H | | | | | | | H | | | | | | | |
| Kinesthetic Differention | H | H | | | | | | | H | H | | | | | | | | | | |

Table 2: Motor abilities developmental periods (adapted from Drabik 1996)

**Practical application of these training principles is very simple. Below are the basic guidelines:**

- For optimal adaptation need to have 2–3 sessions per week

- Many of the exercises can be used as a warm-up
- The exercises are best done when well-rested
- Sessions only need to be 15–30 minutes long

The key is to keep it fun! Whether these exercises are integrated into the warm-up or workout it is best to keep the kids moving the whole time. Intersperse high-level activity with stretching or flexibility rest phases. The following chapter will have examples of workouts and exercises.

**Basic games that can be used are:**

- Simon says
- Follow the leader
- Most number in time
- Relay races

## Speed, Power, and Strength Development in Youth

Development of speed, power, and strength in youth are all neuromuscular-based, hence the same concepts above apply to the development. Many of these drills and exercises overlap, so a drill for rhythm can also be used for power (for example, single leg hops or jumping rope develop rhythm and power, not to mention upper and lower body coordination).

**Speed and power training can develop the following foundation abilities:**

- Limb velocity
- Reaction time
- Frequency of movement
- Improvement in Anaerobic Efficiency

- Amount of glycogen stored in muscles
- Ability to produce energy in the absence of $O_2$
- Ability to perform work when internal environment is disturbed (fatigue, high body temperature, high lactate)

*Table 3: Age-sensitive development ranges (adapted from J. Loko, T. Sikkut, R. Aule)*

| Capacity | Static Strength | Power | | Running Speed |
|---|---|---|---|---|
| | | Legs | Arms | |
| Boys | 13–16 | 13–17 | 13–17 | 12–17 |
| Girls | 11–13 | 10–12 | 10–13 | 10–13 |

*Table 4: Sensitive periods in development of youth motor abilities (adapted from Guzalowski, 1977)*

| Age | 7–8 | | 8–9 | | 9–10 | | 10–11 | | 11–12 | | 12–13 | | 13–14 | | 14–15 | | 15–16 | | 16–17 | |
|---|---|---|---|---|---|---|---|---|---|---|---|---|---|---|---|---|---|---|---|---|
| F-Female M-Male | F | M | F | M | F | M | F | M | F | M | F | M | F | M | F | M | F | M | F | M |
| Absolute Static Strength | L | | L | L | | | H | L | M | | | | | M | | | H | L | | H |
| Speed | H | H | H | H | M | L | H | | | | | | H | | | | L | L | | |
| Speed-Strength | L | | | | H | | H | L | H | | | | L | M | | M | | | | |
| Static Strength Endurance | M | | | | | | H | | M | | H | | | | M | M | H | | | H |

## Strength Training

Strength training in children mainly affects neurogenic mechanisms due to the lack of hormonal support, hence there is no benefit to doing a conventional weight program or the lifting of heavy weights.

The major gains from a body weight-based strength program in youth are:

- Rate coding
- Rate synchronization
- Rate of force development
- Improvement of inter- and intra-muscular coordination

There are many types of strength development. For youth the most important are improvement of muscle balance (development of antagonist and high-risk muscle groups, strengthening of stabilizer, synergist, and neutralizer muscle groups) and core strength. This will provide a great strength base which will reduce the risk of injury no matter what sport the child does later in life.

Incorporating these elements into youth development models will provide a fantastic foundation for any young athlete.

- Juniors ages 6–10 should only do strength training exercises with body weight 15 minutes 3x a week
- Juniors ages 11–14 should focus on strength endurance (intensities no greater than 80% of max) 30 mins 3x a week (Sharkey, 1986)

The exercises used for junior-level training also need to take into account the demands of the other sports that they are doing. For example, female athletes have two times higher of an incidence of non-contact ACL injury in soccer; given this, we need to emphasize development of the glute/hamstring muscle group, medial/lateral stabilizers, as well as the eccentric firing of the quadriceps.

Given a well-designed program one will be able to resist injury as well as progress much quicker in their development as a runner.

## Development of Physiological Base

Most importantly, children need to be active. Having a structured endurance training plan prior to being a J3 has little to no benefit beyond the child having regular physical activity. Regular activity includes being physically active 2–3 days a week and is important for the development of capillarization of muscle tissue, increasing of mitochondrial density, heart stroke volume, and oxygen-carrying capacity. Below one can see some data acquired.

### Endurance Run Until Refusal Tests

| Age | Sex | Training (meters) | NonTraining (meters) | After 1 Year Training (meters) | After 1 Year NonTraining (meters) | After 2 Years Training (meters) | After 2 Years NonTraining (meters) |
|---|---|---|---|---|---|---|---|
| 3 | M | 258 | 254 | 740 | 476 | 1196 | 583 |
| 3 | F | 246 | 235 | 620 | 389 | 1121 | 572 |
| 4 | M | 466 | 460 | 1502 | 622 | 1776 | 716 |
| 4 | F | 370 | 384 | 1146 | 480 | 1479 | 711 |
| 5 | M | 608 | 594 | 1765 | 690 | 2656 | 787 |
| 5 | F | 458 | 452 | 1249 | 676 | 1865 | 786 |

*Table 5: Endurance run to refusal test of youth (adapted from Frolov, Yurko, and Kabachkova, 1974)*

### Endurance Training of Youth Guidelines
- 7–11: 30 mins of endurance training per week, in 5–20 min sections.
- 12–15: 60 mins of endurance training per week in 10–30 min sections.

- When increasing the amount of training, increase volume first, then intensity.

Youth athletes hold a tremendous amount of potential waiting to be expressed and released. As coaches with the proper working knowledge we can act as catalysts to assist and optimize this process. We'd all love to see the children we coach make the Olympics someday, but as youth coaches it is important to realize that we are one step of many in the process of athlete development. Laying a general foundation for the development, enjoyment, and process of training is one of the more important factors in the success in sport. Most importantly, a passion for the process of physical activity needs to be developed; this will come from a fun, dynamic environment that the coach and parents can create.

## Junior Endurance Training

One trap many junior-level runners fall into is doing the majority of their training hours in Level 3. This is a tough habit to break, as we like to encourage runners to train in a group setting. However, the pace often is dictated by the most fit runner's pace that everyone else tries to hang with (who may be in Level 3 or at their level ½ which is everyone else's Levels 3–4). The danger of this continuous moderate training load is the athlete will peak and plateau in six weeks. Given this type of training the athletes will have faster initial fitness gains, but no matter what they do mid-season, they will be stuck at the same lower performance level, relative to an easy-hard periodized loading cycle over the same time where gains will be much greater.

- Development of endurance base and aerobic efficiency (Levels 1–2 training sessions of continuous activity)
- Technique development (dryland drills, basic body position, timing, and weight transfer)
- Core strength

- Strength and power
- Speed (with high quality technique)

Guidelines for Annual Training Hours (USST) Age 16: 350–400

- Age 17: 400–500
- Age 18: 450–550
- Age 19: 550+
- Age 20: 650+
- Age 21: 700+

# 5

# Testing and Evaluation

## Introduction

Runner performance evaluation is one of the most important factors in the development of a training program. The purpose is to give the athlete a baseline of their performance, data to set specific goals, then monthly (or more frequently) spot testing will give them metrics on their performance gains. Most importantly, it is valuable feedback on if the training plan is working as planned.

Based on initial athlete evaluation, an athlete is able to start the planning process with specific goals. They will have an objective, individualized profile of their strengths and weaknesses. This baseline is the foundation from which we work and determine what type of training will be most beneficial to an individual athlete.

All of the best training plans in the world are useless if the individual athlete's evaluation is not done. Without it, the athlete does not objectively know if the training stimulus has the expected and desired outcome. Is the athlete a responder or non-responder to the training stimulus? How do you fine-tune for that individual? Evaluation allows one to systematically alter training variables and determine objectively if the adaptation has been achieved. Many experienced coaches have the ability or sense to ascertain this from daily contact with the athlete. Objective measurements offer exact data on changes in performance.

Another important factor is the management of the training data. With the evolution of high-quality GPS-based training watches, training data can easily be quantified, recorded, and uploaded to an online database. This is the most effective method to manage the training data.

## How to Test

For accessibility, efficiency, accuracy, and ease of use, field tests are the most effective and efficient means of evaluation. They require minimal equipment and time and can be done in a group setting, which is ideal for coaches. Field tests are very effective in measuring specific elements of performance. Years ago, as new physiologists, we were very focused on lab-based testing of endurance athletes. While this has value, it is not practical or economical for developing junior and master-level athletes. A physical exam should be conducted first, and if the athlete is cleared by their physician for physical activity, the next step is to have a Functional Movement or Original Strength Screen. This is a robust tool in predicting injury risk and very useful in evaluating kinetic chain balance or lack thereof.

Lastly we can get into full-throttle performance testing, of endurance, speed, strength and power.

The evaluation of an athlete's training capacity can be divided into five categories: medical; functional movement/kinetic chain evaluation; aerobic, strength, and power performance; aerobic/anaerobic efficiency; and lactate testing.

**Medical Evaluation**

Medical evaluation is critical prior to starting any physical fitness program. The physician is responsible for administering the medical assessment of the athlete's health status and giving his permission for further participation in an exercise program. The reason for this is to avoid exacerbation of any pre-existing medical condition and early diagnosis of any health problem that will jeopardize the athlete's safety prior to starting physical fitness performance measurements or regularly scheduled exercise workouts.

**Evaluating the Kinetic Chain**

FMS (functional movement screens) and Original Strength movement Screens are a global method of assessment of an athlete's muscle balance, mobility, and stability. A score of less than 14 (out of a possible 21) on the FMS is a highly predictive indicator of sports injury risk. This is especially relevant in runners who have recurrent injuries. There are a number of tests that are very helpful to the coach to determine if the athlete has any injury risk factors or core/stabilization strength imbalances that will affect the runner's ability to optimize their body position and technique. Every runner will benefit from this testing as it will also give insights on how to improve running efficiency. Imagine gaining 4-6 inches of stride length off of improved mobility! This could yield an 4-6 minute decrease in one's 10k time. This is best evaluated by a trainer or coach who is FMS or OS certified. The test takes about 30 minutes.

## Running-Specific Performance Testing

### 5,000/1,500-Meter Running Test

Protocol: This test is performed on a track. The athlete is timed for 5,000 meters (Obtain split times at every 1,000 meters; this can indicate an athlete's ability to pace well (and determine if they went out too fast or too slow for an optimal time). Break for two hours, then run 1,500 meters for time.

### Lactate Testing

Lactate testing is the gold standard for quantifying individual training zones. The test correlates lactate levels to specific work output levels based upon other measurable variables like heart rate, speed, or power output (watts). This allows the runner to determine their individualized training zones and get a baseline to boot. If six months later you are running 1,000 meters at a faster speed, lower HR, and lower lactate level for the same time/speed, then you know you had a performance improvement. What makes lactate so important is that it helps the runner determine the metabolic bottlenecks in their performance and target their training more effectively. For example, runner A may need to spend more time doing Level 1 and 2 training over the summer, whereas Runner B may need to do more Level 4 intervals.

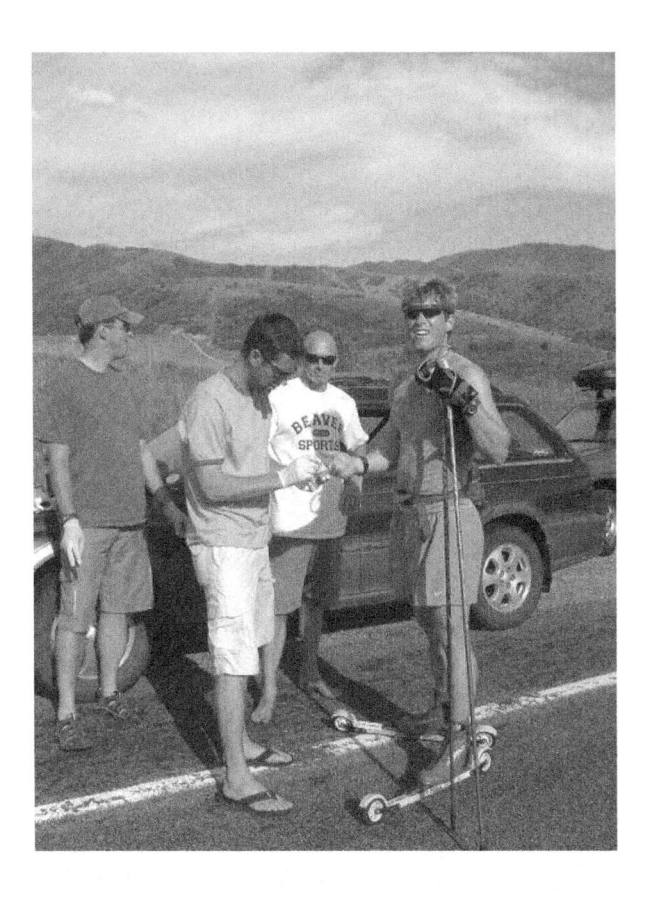

## Background

The basis for lactate testing comes from the area called bioenergetics or energy systems. This is the process of how the body takes fuel and converts it to energy or work. To do this, our body has three primary energy systems that are constantly working together in different proportions. This is kind of like a hybrid car where, when it is driving in traffic, it uses electricity, and when it accelerates, it uses both electricity and gas, and when it is on the highway, it uses only gas. Our body has a similar process. Our body uses different energy systems and different proportions of energy systems for different durations and intensities of exercise.

## ATP-PC System

For short duration (4–10 seconds) or very high-intensity exercise (like sprinting 60 to 100 meters), our body uses the ATP-PC system.

## Glycolysis

Used for exercise at a high intensity or lasting 45–60 seconds.

## Aerobic System

Used for easy to moderate intensity levels and durations of exercise of 1 minute to 3 hours.

Imagine that you are starting your afternoon run. No matter what speed you start at, for the first 8–10 seconds, you are using your ATP-PC energy system. The ATP-PC system uses ATP and phospho-creatine that is in the muscle tissue for the first bit of energy. After this, it starts to be depleted, and the body then switches over to glycolysis. This gives us another 45–60 seconds of energy, but since this is not an aerobic system, the byproduct is the production of lactate or hydrogen ions (H+), which no one likes, especially us aerobic athletes.

After 40–60 seconds (given the intensity is easy to moderate), you switch over now to your aerobic system where you are metabolizing glycogen and fat stored in your muscle tissue and liver. If your intensity increases beyond a certain level or you run out of glycogen, say you are running up a hill, or you have been running for 3.5 hours, your energy system proportions again switch over to glycolysis being the dominant system. With well-trained/conditioned athletes, their bodies (through training/adaptation) deal with lactate in three ways. One, they function aerobically at a higher work level and don't produce as much lactate at a given work level. Two, they buffer lactate very effectively, so when they produce it, the body processes it and neutralizes it very quickly so it has little adverse effect. Three, when they produce lactate, they have adapted to tolerate very high levels while still maintaining good technique and power output.

The lactate that is a byproduct of glycolysis is acidic, which interferes with all sorts of our physical operations. Our stomach does not like the acid; hence, we feel nauseous. Our muscle tissue cannot carry on its metabolic processes in this acidic environment, so the muscles stop functioning, and our nervous system cannot function. Eventually, since the nerves have impaired firing, we first lose coordination at lower levels of acidosis. At higher levels, our nerves just stay on, and our muscle keeps firing, which is cramping—even more fun!

Lactate is a byproduct of an energy system that we start to use when we are exceeding our aerobic capabilities. It is a great marker to measure our aerobic and anaerobic fitness.

## Purpose of Lactate Testing

Lactate is one of several measurements of aerobic physiological performance. Other measurements are $VO_2$ max and max heart rate. Lactate is the most accurate standard by which to measure an individual's performance because it gives a very accurate physiological measurement of one's aerobic and anaerobic work output. When we test lactate, we are looking for a graph of data points, some in a "steady state" of exercise below 4 mmol, which is at a level that you can exercise for several hours at an aerobic level. Then, we also are looking for data points and their progression above 4 mmol. This is at a point where we are no longer functioning aerobically, and so we have a finite amount of time (depending upon the lactate level) of how long we can exercise before our muscles stop functioning. At higher and higher intensity levels, lactate increases, and the amount of time we can stay at this higher intensity decreases.

## Lactate Testing Protocol

Have athlete warm-up in level 1 for 10 minutes. Make sure they do not get out of this range as it will confound testing results.

Have the athlete run or run a set loop (ideally on a track) at a constant heart rate for 5 minutes. As soon as they return, sample lactate, record data, then have athlete progress to next exertion level to repeat the test.

The first test the athlete should start in their predicted (by percentage of maximum heart rate, as a basic guideline) level 1. Each consecutive test should be at a progressively higher exertion level (1–5). I highly recommend reviewing the data off the monitor post test to make sure the athlete was in the correct level. Often times spurious results are due to the athlete yo-yoing their lactate levels, i.e. jumping into level 5 for 1 minute then dropping down to level 3, which will result in a higher lactate level that is not a realistic representation of their true HR based values.

**GM Lactate Testing**

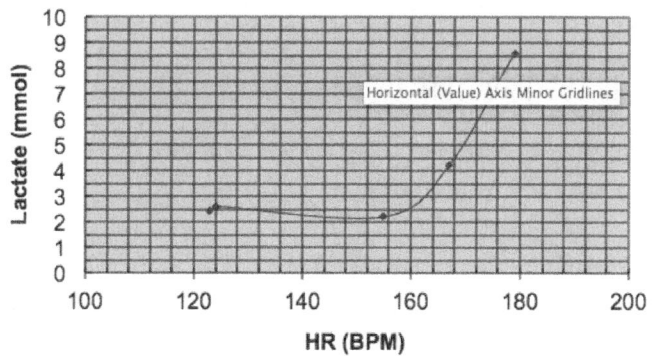

*Graph 2: Lactate testing curve of HR and lactate*

## What the Numbers Mean

4 mmol of lactate is the magic number for most athletes. Below this, athletes are at a steady state of exercise (i.e., one is

functioning fully aerobically and not producing much lactate, so they can continue exercising for three or more hours). Above 4 mmol/L of lactate one's body is switching over to using energy systems that are producing lactate at a higher rate than the body can buffer it. Hence at higher and higher levels of work above 4 mmol/L one has a finite amount of time they can perform at this work level, because they are accumulating more and more lactate. As a point of reference, elite runners routinely race with lactate levels of 13–16 mmol/L. This is part of what makes them "elite" in their capability to manage and perform at those lactate levels.

**Time Trials**

Fast, functional, relevant performance evaluation. Time trials are an excellent method of routine testing to evaluate the effectiveness of your training. When doing a time trial it is important that it is as standardized as possible on the same course or track.

- Use the same route/track each time testing
- Ideally test same time of day

## Putting the Tests to Work for You

You have completed most or all of your evaluation. What does it mean, and what do you change in your training?

First and foremost address mobility/stability deficits, and injury risk factors related to strength or muscle imbalances. This should be your priority. It is not good judgment to continue training only to take 3-6 weeks off to treat a preventable injury. Injuries should not be viewed as a badge of honor of pushing hard. It is only clear evidence of a poorly designed and ineffectively implemented training program.

If you are training six hours a week, the majority of your time (3–4 hours) should be focused on addressing these deficits so you have a strong foundation to build the rest of your training on. This time may seem like you are going backward on your running-specific fitness but it will pay huge dividends in improved sport performance and injury resistance. In most cases, with 2–3 weeks' time with a good maintenance program, your deficits will be improved to the point that you can resume focused training.

Once injury risk factors are addressed start with looking at what your goals are relative to your competitive timeline. If you are six months out from your peak race then you have time to periodize your training to meet most of your goals. If you are just 2–3 months out then you need to really prioritize the biodynamic elements that you can effectively change in a short period of time. These are strength, power, technique, and—to a limited degree—peak aerobic performance. Aerobic endurance adaptations take many months to change significantly. If you have the goal of racing a marathon, and you have had minimal aerobic volume training, you may have to adjust your goal or timeline for that goal.

For overall training planning guidelines, refer back to the training planning chapter.

# 6

# Overtraining

## Too Much of a Good Thing

As the demands of competitive sports are becoming greater, recovery from training and competition has become even more important to prevent overtraining. Recovery is physiological as well psychological. In other words, recovery is a generic term used specifically in reference to the restoration of physiological and psychological states that have been excessively stressed or altered during a particular activity (Yessis, 1982).

Training for Running relies on a high load (intensity and volume) of exercise that will induce significant changes in the athlete's body. These changes are extremely important for performance improvement. However, if training stress exceeds the athlete's capacity to recover between training stimuli, a significant amount of fatigue will accumulate. The accumulation of fatigue is more likely responsible for the lack of training progress. Overreaching is short-term fatigue that can last over 1–2 weeks. During times of increased volume loading during camps or during an intensity block phase this imbalance of adaptation is an expected finding. However, if the athlete continues to remain fatigued greater than two weeks and is not tolerating their normal training load, they have moved into a more advanced condition. Overtraining is prolonged fatigue lasting greater than two weeks.

Prolonged fatigue (overtraining syndrome), or so-called long-term fatigue, is associated with peripheral and "central" fatigue (Lehmann et al., 1993).

It is important to remember that this is an imbalance between training load and regeneration. The imbalance can be developed by inadequate regeneration or additional stresses that add into physiological, endocrinological, or psychological stress such as impaired sleep; stress at work or school; emotional stress due to personal, work, or family relationships; or physical illness.

The primary types of fatigue are neuromuscular, metabolic, and neuroendocrine.

## Neuromuscular Fatigue

Our neuromuscular system consists of our peripheral and central nervous system. Our peripheral nervous system consists of our motor neurons and neural pathways from the spinal column. Every time we move a muscle we are firing our motor neurons; when we are doing high motor skill or physical intensity activities we are stressing this system at its highest level. Our motor neurons and sensory motor system are hit with a double whammy of stress. The first is from the metabolic wastes produced by muscular metabolism and tissue damage. The second is the physiological stress on the motor neuron itself (ion channels/membranes, electrolyte changes, and metabolic stress of the cells themselves). To add further complications, our neuromuscular system has much less blood perfusion than our muscle tissue and relies on axonal transport to remove metabolic wastes and transport regenerative nutrients. This regenerative process takes 2–3 times longer than our muscles: 36–72 hours. Net result neuromuscular overtraining is much more likely to occur in athletes. The initial symptoms are insidious, as they are not easy to recognize, but they have a significant negative impact on our performance.

Krestovnikov (1951) proposed that it takes a nervous cell seven times as long to recover than a skeletal muscle cell. This is due to the slow rate of recovery of the motor neuron units that recruit a given muscle. This has implications with how one organizes training and how much of a taper an athlete needs to recover sufficiently before optimal performance. If the athlete is not fully recovered neurophysiologically, coordination, force production, and balance will be impaired. As coaches we often do not notice poor neuromuscular recovery in the beginning of the season. However, towards the end of the season, we often see very fit athletes have poor performances; this is due to impaired force production and fine motor skill coordination, the factors that make an athlete efficient. The next question is how do we accelerate the recovery of the motor neuron units? So far the best method is rest. To date there has been little research in this area, though due to the increased understanding of the importance of the neuromuscular system, this is an area of increasing interest.

The neuromuscular load is one of the most stressful. The high intensity training work in the yearly cycle leads to significant fatigue of the athlete's entire body. During the time of hard training, both the entire muscular system and the supporting neuro-motor system become very fatigued. This process has an impact on executing dynamic movements that require a high range of motion (flexibility) and coordination (Paikov V.B, 1985). The rate at which an athlete recovers from any sources of fatigue or exhaustion determines the rate at which training can progress.

Besides the peripheral muscular fatigue, which is primarily biochemical in nature, the athlete also can experience a more powerful syndrome of fatigue of the CNS (Central Nervous System). In running, with a high intensity, the CNS is fatigued due to the extremely high rate of motor neurons firing. CNS fatigue is reached when one's training has sent too many strong stimuli within a short time frame. Therefore the neuromuscular system is not able to produce a maximum contraction of the muscle, and loss of velocity may begin. This negative change occurs when the byproducts of high intensity running (speed) build up to the point where CNS impulses cannot sufficiently stimulate fast twitch muscle fibers to contract.

The CNS has to be fully regenerated so that the chemical environment (sodium/potassium balance and removal of waste products) required for optimal transmission of nervous signal is intact.

**Symptoms of Neuromuscular Fatigue**

- Decreased maximal power output
- Decreased fine motor coordination (think decreased balance, coordination, timing, and loss of proprioception in running)
- Decreased maximal speed
- Reduction in velocity of consecutive repetitions
- Reduction of athlete's ability to demonstrate proper running form (lower hip position, leaning posture)
- Lack of relaxation during activity

Given this higher level of fatigue our recovery may be required far beyond the initial Petrovski's rest interval stages time, especially during the over-speed training.

**The CNS Needs Additional Time to Regenerate**
This can be done by:

- Extension of time of rest interval to 3 minutes
- Higher number of sets
- Low number of repetition in set (maximum 3)
- Active rest between sets
- 80% simple technical drills; the application of these drills will help us to maximize the adaptation level toward the next set

An incomplete recovery of muscular motor units requires an increase in nerve stimulation and recruitment of additional motor neuron units resulting in increased oxygen requirements (Lehmann et al., 1993). Incomplete recovery and premature fatigue of motor units may be based partly on the reduction of muscular glycogen reserves and phosphocreatine, or on the accumulation of protons, whereas an additional decrease in hepatic glycogen and blood glucose level promote central and peripheral fatigue (Lehmann et al., 1993). This transition from short-term to long-term fatigue is smooth and continuous if stressors are maintained without proper recovery.

# Metabolic Fatigue

Metabolic fatigue is related to our muscular system. Exercise at any level induces stress on our muscles. With long endurance workouts muscles fatigue due to accumulated metabolic waste. High intensity (interval and speed) workouts contract more muscle tissue and accumulating higher levels of hydrogen ions, which damage muscle tissue (and motor neuron units). If we repeat high level stresses on our muscles they too will not adequately regenerate. Under optimal conditions our muscles regenerate in 12–24 hours.

Symptoms of metabolic fatigue are:

- Increased muscle soreness
- Increased fatigue at easy levels of exercise
- Increased resting heart rate (greater than 10% for two days or more)
- Increased generalized fatigue, lack of motivation to train

## Neuroendocrine Fatigue

Neuroendocrine fatigue is related to our hormonal response to exercise and stress. With physical activity we secrete epinephrine, norepinephrine, human growth hormones (HGH), thyroid-stimulating hormones, and cortisol (Bompa, 1999). With high levels of physical activity or generalized stress, we can deplete (or have hormonal imbalances) which result in a decreased ability to adapt.

**Symptoms of Neuroendocrine Fatigue**
- Impaired ability to sleep
- Increased resting heart rate (greater than 10% for two days or more)
- Increased depression/melancholy
- Decreased concentration
- Increased risk of infection

It is especially important to note that the immune response is suppressed for 3–72 hours after high intensity exercise. In the case of competitions, athletes need to pay special attention to this and not come in close contact with people that are sick in order to avoid risk of infection, which could result in setbacks in training and performance (Hoffman and Peterson, 1994).

The well-conditioned athlete should almost fully recover within 12–24 hours after an intense training session. However, an athlete may not have sufficient time to fully recuperate if the next training session is scheduled too soon after the previous session, or regeneration is impaired by additional stresses (impaired sleep, emotional, or school stress). Sometimes the purpose of the next intense training workout is to stimulate a stronger adaptation of a given system (such as that in intensity blocks). That results in a performance increase of the next training session if the training session only includes similar physiological stresses. For conventional intensity training loads, another, similar type of workout can be resumed after 48 to 56 hours of resting period.

*Table 6: Over-reached athlete: Markers and parameters of temporary fatigue (adapted from Lee, 2000). Source: Lehmann et al. (1993)*

| Possible Mediators of the Over-reached response | |
|---|---|
| Neural Fatigue | Altered Immune Status |
| Decreased Work Capacity | Increased Sympathetic Tone |
| Glycogen Depletion | Reduced O2 Transport Capacity |
| Decreased Efficiency of Movement | Slower Onset of Anabolic |
| Cell Membrane/Organelle Damage | Reactions Following Exercise |

Short-term overtraining, or overreaching, may result in imbalances in the body's functional systems, which in turn are reflected by the expression of changes in measurable markers. Recognition of these markers may enable training to be reduced before the overtraining syndrome (Fry et al., 1992).

## Prolonged Fatigue or Possibilities of Overtraining

If sufficient rest is not included in a training program then regeneration cannot occur and performance plateaus. If this imbalance between excess training and inadequate rest persists then performance will decline. The other causes of overtraining syndrome are excessive amounts of high intensity training accumulated in short periods of time between 2–3 weekly microcycles. The athlete's body is not capable of adapting to a sudden increase of training load, and the adaptation process is temporarily shut down.

Therefore, prolonged fatigue or overtraining can best be defined as the state where the athlete has been repeatedly stressed by training to the point where rest is no longer adequate to allow for recovery. The "overtraining syndrome" is the name given to the collection of emotional, behavioral, and physical symptoms due to overtraining that has persisted from weeks to months (Jenky, 1999).

There have been several clinical studies conducted on athletes showing prolonged fatigue and overtraining syndrome. Most of these studies included extensive physiological, psychological, and biochemical laboratory exercise testing. In most cases these tests have shown significantly decreased performance in exercise testing, decreased mood state, and, in some, increased cortisol levels (the body's "stress" hormone). A decrease in testosterone, altered immune status, and an increase in muscular breakdown products have also been identified (Jenky, 1999).

The breakdown products of protein metabolism, such as ammonia and urea, have accumulated when athletes exceeded their base metabolic scores and start utilizing muscular protein tissue as an energy source. After hard training the blood levels rise and unwanted metabolism waste products damage cells that release enzymes such as creatine kinase. The ratio of testosterone to cortisol is used as an indication of the buildup and breakdown of tissue. As tissue is broken down and the stress on the body increases, testosterone levels go down and cortisol levels rise. When your body is exhausted, blood levels of the stress hormones, adrenaline and noradrenaline, rise. Blood levels drop of ACTH which stimulates your adrenal glands, growth hormone, cortisol, and insulin (Jenky, 1999).

*Table 7: Physiological and psychological symptoms and signs of overtraining (adapted from Calder, 1993)*

| PHYSIOLOGICAL | PSYCHOLOGICAL |
|---|---|
| 1. Elevated resting HR | 1. Disturbed sleep |
| 2. Decreased weight | 2. Poor motivation |
| 3. Increased muscle soreness/tenderness | 3. Irritability |
| 4. Increased fatigue | 4. Depression |
| 5. Increased blood lactate | 5. Increased anxiety |
| 6. Decreased nerve impulse transmission | 6. Increased nervousness |
| 7. Decreased aerobic threshold | 7. Increased fatigue |
| 8. Increased anaerobic threshold | 8. Decreased vigor |
| 9. Increased susceptibility to illness | 9. Depressed mood state |
| 10. Tendency to headaches, colds, and fever blisters | 10. Decline in feelings of self-worth |
| 11. Decreased appetite | 11. Uncontrollable emotions |
| 12. Elevated blood pressure | 12. Insecurity |
| 13. Decreased energy levels | 13. Oversensitive about criticism |
| 14. Increased fatigue = lower tolerance of workload | 14. Listlessness |
| 15. Increased muscle tension | 15. Melancholy |
| 16. Impaired coordination and reaction time | |
| 17. Night sweats | |
| 18. Higher breathing rate under normal physical stress | |
| 19. Prolonged recovery time between workouts | |

Under normal circumstances there is a balance between the autonomic nervous system and endocrine system. In the overtrained state, the normal homeostasis balance is disturbed and the athlete experiences a temporary disruption of the body's normal biological function-rhythm. Therefore, medically speaking, the overtraining syndrome is classified as a neuro-endocrine disorder. In this state the athlete will feel fatigued, depressed/melancholy, be at higher risk of infection (or have symptoms of a low-level cold), and/or have a loss of motivation. Female athletes at this point will have delayed (or loss of) menses.

Prolonged fatigue should be viewed as a continuum process from where the athlete is optimally recuperated after a training overload to extremely overtrained. The continuum process of overtraining is best describe as the circling process.

*Figure 1: The circling process of overtraining syndrome (adapted from Traeger and Hooper, 1993)*

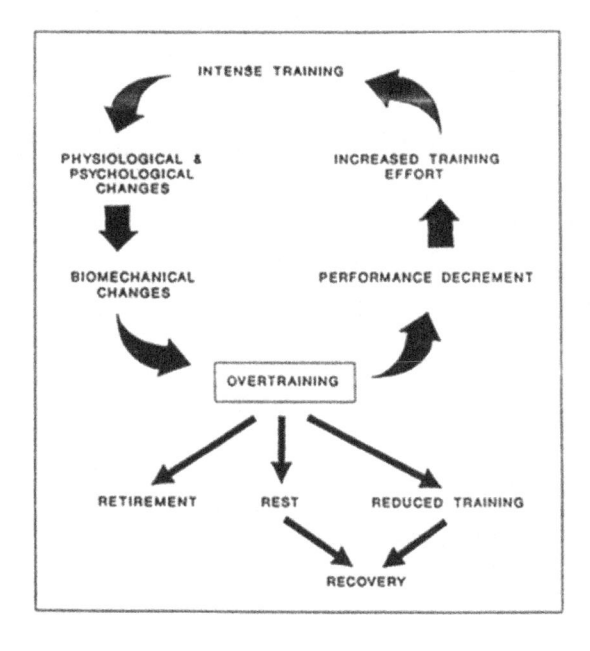

The earliest signs of overtraining are neuromuscular-based (disruption of neuromuscular coordination, decreased power output, and snap/precision of movement) even though a classic overtrained state has not been reached (Calder, 1993). The physiological and psychological symptoms of overtraining are often the later indicators of overtraining.

Improper interpretation of a temporary decline of performance due to insufficient implementation of recovery time and regeneration modalities often are misinterpreted by the athlete as not being trained enough even though the opposite is the truth. This decline in performance often forces the athlete to train harder. The increased training effort will intensify and prolong fatigue, which may be recognized as overtraining syndrome. Increasing number of workouts onto this unbalanced system only worsens the situation. The circle of overtraining will continue to spiral, and the athlete's body now has a decreased ability to recover itself during rest. This will significantly affect one's ability to continue to train and compete on a high level (Hooper et al, 1993).

## Avoidance of Overtraining Syndrome

The possibility of overtraining syndrome has been a major concern in training methodology for decades. In recent years it is even more important since training loads have increased to the point where each training session is finished on the edge of excessive fatigue.

Physiologic improvement in training only occur during the rest period following sufficient overloading of cardiovascular and neuromuscular systems. The athlete's adaptation to the training stimulus represents an improvement in the cardiovascular system by increasing capillaries and mitochondrial enzymes, improved neuromuscular coordination by better synchronization of muscle contractions, and increased glycogen stores within the muscle cells. During the recovery period the utilized components of these systems are rebuilt and adapt to exceed the initial level (supercompensation), so the result is that the athlete reaches a higher level of training capacity.

**Proper Periodization of Recovery Process**

Running relies heavily on well-designed training periodization. In periodized training the load varies in cycles and is directly connected to an annual plan. Some cycles are of high overload, where others represent moderate stimulation. The high workload phase will bring the required adaptation, but must be scheduled well and planned out. Hard work requires sufficient recovery and alternation of the training stimuli. In this approach a yearly training schedule must take into account a plan that includes predicted periods of decreased training load (intensity and volume) as a precaution to avoid exhaustion.

From exercise physiology of sports training we know that any performance improvement is possible where the adaptation process has occurred and reached a maximum level. After that the performance will reach stagnation (plateau) and finally start to decline. In order to avoid the stagnation and bring our athlete to even higher levels of adaptation to new training stimuli, planning and recovery must be introduced.

*Table 8: Objectives of recovery process in yearly periodized training programs*

Athletes must make strenuous efforts toward a higher level of adaptation and enter the zone of an excessive fatigue state. At this point the regeneration process (reduction of training stimuli) becomes necessary. The stronger the overtraining state, the longer amount of rest is required. Therefore, early rectification of training exhaustion must be a major goal of proper training planning .

If the physiological overtraining is for a short period of time, no more than 3–4 weekly microcycles, an unloading recovery microcycle must be introduced. When a training period of intense training exceeds six weeks, a few unloading microcycles alternated with maximum loading will prevent overload and maladaptation.

The unloading microcycle has decreased volume, however the intensity level is maintained, with lower volume. For example, if you are normally doing 4 x 5-minute intervals you would decrease the time to 4 minutes or decrease the number of repetitions so the total time in Level 5 decreases from 20 minutes to 12–15 minutes. The best indicator of when to decrease your interval training load is interval performance. If your HR is drifting out of range, or for the same time and distance on the same interval course, and you are going a shorter and shorter distance with the same intensity of effort, then it is time to stop the workout.

If the athlete has reached current adaptation (maximum exercise capacity), a reduction of about 20–25% of present training load, with a change in the exercise mode (switch from running to nordic skiing, or rowing at a lower intensity level), should eliminate the plateau, and recover the athlete to the level where they are able to achieve a new adaptation. There is considerable evidence that reduced training (same intensity, lower volume) for up to 21 days will not decrease performance. The alternate day recovery period is continued for a few weeks and then an increase in volume is permitted. In more severe cases, the training program may have to be interrupted for weeks, and it may take months to recover. An alternate form of exercise can be substituted to help prevent the exercise withdrawal syndrome (Jenky, 1999).

# 7

# Regeneration Strategies for Optimizing Adaptation

## Introduction

Optimal training adaptation is a balance between training load and regeneration. For many years physiologists' primary focus was on the training load component and periodization process. However, we realized that this had limitations. If the athlete could not adapt to the training load, they became fatigued then overtrained—an imbalance between load and regeneration. With optimal regeneration, runners can tolerate a higher training load and have even more rapid adaptations. Imagine if we could compress two years of training into one. We could make immense gains! However, we have found there are finite boundaries of how quickly one can regenerate. This chapter will discuss the process of regenerative strategies review that are effective in accelerating the adaptation process.

According to Calder (1993), the regeneration process refers to and athlete's return to baseline physiological and psychological parameters; excessive or prolonged training increases risk of injury and decreases resistance of immune system of an athlete's body.

I have always told my athletes recovery starts *prior* to training, not just after training. If you start your race or training already in the hole you will just have that much more to climb out of to achieve optimal recovery.

Prior to the workout you want to be well-rested, hydrated, and fueled—this will go a long way to feeling good and getting the most out of the session. I find with high school athletes this is an area in need of high improvement, sometimes due to inattention, other times logistics . All schools and most workplaces have climate-controlled ventilation that dehumidifies the air, which further increases the need for extra hydration.

Dehydration is an insidious factor on performance. At a 1% decrease in bodyweight due to water loss the body is starting to have performance decreases. This is the point where you are feeling thirsty. At a 4% decrease there is a 20–30% decrease in exercise performance. If you usually run a 36-minute 10k you will be coming in at 43–46 minutes (Grandjean & Ruud, 1994)!

At this point I am going to make my disclosure and recommend specific products for regeneration. I have been sponsored by Hammer Nutrition, and know those products best after 20 years of trying a variety of other brand products (many have come and gone). These have worked best for me, however, everybody is built differently, so there is some trial and error to see what products work best for you. At least this will provide a starting point for you to understand the key ingredients that go into developing a good product and you can make your decision from there.

## The Everyday Basics of Regeneration That Matter Most

### Be Well-Hydrated and Fueled Prior to Training and Competition

Water is the best fluid to drink to be well-hydrated over the course of the day. Just prior to and during competition you can switch to a balanced product that has some electrolytes and complex carbohydrates (maltodextrin). For this Hammer Nutrition HEED can be very effective. An important part of what helps you stay hydrated is gastric emptying rate. Nutritionists have found that straight water does not empty as rapidly (i.e., get circulated systemically as quickly as water with complex sugars). The electrolytes will also help with keeping your sodium, potassium, and calcium in balance so you will be less likely to cramp with extended exercise at a race pace.

### Warm-Up

**Start exercise with a good warm-up.** Our gym teachers weren't lying when they tried to teach us to warm up well. The research on warming up and injury prevention is abundant; without it, your risk of injury skyrockets. I recommend starting with myofascial release (i.e., rolling out with a foam roller or rolling stick), then go into some diaphragmatic breathing exercises with active/dynamic range of motion activity (rolling, rocking, crawling, cross crawls). These specific exercises are called re-sets (and will be discussed in my other book) and they serve to improve your mobility, core strength, and neuromuscular reactivity (balance, quickness, reactive strength). Then start your specific activity for the day, keep your heart rate in Levels 1–2 for the first 5–7 minutes, then you can progress from there. If you are doing an intensity workout add in 3–5, 5-second sprints to increase your heart rate to prepare for the first intervals.

**During the workout or race.** Continue to be well-hydrated. You should be drinking 150ml every 15 minutes, then up to 300ml every 15 minutes in hot weather. For workouts over an hour, strongly consider a drink with electrolytes and carbohydrates to replenish fuels as you train. For workouts over two hours, the drink should have protein in addition to carbohydrates and electrolytes.

## Warm-Down

If you are doing a long, easy run in Levels 1–2 then you are pretty well set with no warm-down. If you did an interval or speed workout, a 10–15 minute warm-down in Levels 1–2 is critical to flush out the metabolic waste in your muscle tissue. Without the warm-down you will have residual muscle soreness and delayed regeneration.

Once your warm-down is complete you have a 10- to 15-minute window for optimal hydration and supplementation for regeneration. This is a critical time frame to rehydrate and replenish your muscles with carbohydrate, protein amino acids, and electrolytes. Every hour you wait to replenish these, your recovery decreases by a significant amount. This transfers to being already in the hole the next day for your next workout. For this I have utilized Hammer Nutrition's Recoverite.

In order to achieve the best possible training effect either physiologically or psychologically the recovery process must focus on the following aspects:

- The removal of accumulated lactate products from working muscles
- The overcoming of high muscle tension (very often muscle spasm)
- The replenishment of body fuel stores

- The restoration of muscle tissue, which was stressed during high intensity training
- Regeneration of CNS

From sport physiology, we know that recovery time is different for speed, strength, power, or even endurance. Therefore, the time required for recovery of different biodynamic characteristics varies a great deal as does the time for the replenishment of biochemical energy sources. However, the replacement of creatine phosphate (CP) reserve is very fast. The replacement of glycogen and the mending of damaged muscle elements takes much longer as does the regeneration of the motor neurons.

Multiple consecutive high intensity days utilizes the anaerobic alactic and lactic energy system using glycogen as fuel. Without the possibility of replenishing the depleted fuel and regeneration of the CNS, this will significantly reduce one's ability to perform effectively during and immediately after each training session.

The scheduling of recovery modalities is important and individualized to suit the particular athlete's adaptability, work capacity, and recuperative powers, as well as the demands of the sport. Therefore, the athlete's entire cardiovascular and neuromuscular system needs time to adapt to:

- Workload = Overcompensation
- Overcompensation = Adaptive Response
- Recovery = Essential for Adaptation

**Sleep for Regeneration**

Sleep is one of the most important things athletes can do for optimal regeneration. The active body needs 9–10 hours of sleep each night. Studies have found that inadequate sleep results in a higher injury rate and decreased athletic performance. This is even more important for junior-level athletes where it is recommended to have 9–10 hours of sleep a night. For many junior-level runners this is often neglected, especially given the distraction of electronic devices. When we sleep not only does our brain rest, but our body repairs itself. Hormonally, we secrete growth hormones which aid in the regeneration process, and sleep is critical for rapid CNS regeneration. If athletes find they are having difficulty sleeping then adding in breathing exercises and meditation earlier in their day can help reduce stress and anxiety that is impairing sleep.

**Periodized Rest Days**

An important step in prevention of overtraining is to structure training plans to include rest days during microcycles and unloading weeks in microcycles to accommodate adaptation and promote supercompensation.

## Regeneration Modalities

The athlete's adaptation to a training load involves repetitive stress of major systems in order to stimulate physiological responses, even though the training stimulus can differ in degree of magnitude and the specificity of work. Planning rest periods between training stimuli or training sessions is a necessary part of any well-designed training program. Well-organized and balanced training structures must take into consideration all principles and modalities of training recovery. Application of these vital principals will help recognize and avoid overtraining as soon as it is detected and decrease the chance of prolonged exhaustion and overtraining.

*Table 9: The main objectives and methods of sport training recovery modalities (adapted from Matuszewski, 1992)*

| Recovery Modalities | Main Objectives and Methods |
|---|---|
| Work/rest ratios | 1. Active rest<br>2. Active rest |
| Hydro Therapy | 1. Bath/showers<br>2. Float tanks (flotation)<br>3. Contrasting temperature— hot/cold<br>4. Sauna (dry baths) |
| Sport Massage | 1. Therapeutic massage<br>2. Localized massage<br>3. Underwater massage |
| Acupressure/ Acupuncture | 1. Pain relief<br>2. Muscle relaxation (increase band straining) |
| Use of heat | 1. Dry heat (ultraviolet irradiation, infrared light)<br>2. Moist heat (paraffin wax, mud baths) |
| Electrotherapy | 1. Electronic Muscle Stimulation (EMS)<br>2. Magnetic Interferential Laser<br>3. Galvanization<br>4. Diathermy |

| Psychotherapy | |
|---|---|
| | 1. Stress management<br>2. Relaxation training |
| Nutrition | |
| | 1. Water<br>2. Vitamins and minerals<br>3. Supplements and ergogenic aids |

The process of early detection of overtraining syndrome is the responsibility of both the coach and the athlete.

## Responsibility of the Coach

- Teach athlete signs and symptoms of overtraining
- Plan recovery regimen
- Familiarize athletes with recovery modalities and reinforce regularly
- Monitor athletes for overtraining signs and symptoms
- Adjust recovery regimen according to workloads, environmental constraints, individual needs

## Responsibility of the Athlete

- Learn signs and symptoms of overtraining
- Monitor for early signs of overreaching and communicate to coach
- Become familiar with recovery areas/modalities
- Become responsible for administering these as effectively as possible

The best method to monitor all physiological and psychological changes of an athlete's state is a training log. In most cases athletes use a log-book for monitoring of training load; application of training stimuli; type, volume, and intensity of exercises; break between exercises; or time between the next training session.

The coach must keep track of all training parameters in order to control the training process. Very seldom do athletes go above the standard monitoring. The athlete should provide for the coach resting heart rate, body weight, quality of sleep, magnitude of soreness, attitude toward new workout, general aspect of nutrition and health symptoms, and general overview of how they feel. This will make it possible to modify the current program in order to avoid overtraining.

## Work/Rest Ratios, Including Light Post-Workout Active Recovery

The primary treatment for any type of fatigue from physical activities is properly executed rest. In order to improve athlete physiological responses to adaptation, sufficient time of active and passive rest must be planned. The systematic inclusion of active and passive recovery sessions reduce overtraining and possibilities of injury.

Regeneration will depend upon the type of recovery (active recovery or passive recovery) and level of fatigue incurred, the energy system involved in training session (anaerobic, alactic, or lactic), type of training session (strength, speed, plyometrics, or interval), and training phase (preparation or competition).

*Table 10: Modalities of active and passive rest after training sessions (adapted from Recovery and Regeneration, compiled articles for the International Coaching School, Victoria, BC, Canada, 1993)*

| REST PROCESS | |
|---|---|
| ACTIVE REST | PASSIVE REST |
| Lighter activities at the end of session | Do nothing |
| Stretching after each workload/session | Proper sleep |
| Lighter aerobic work after session<br>• Walk<br>• Jog<br>• Cycle<br>• Swim | Monitoring of major body<br>• Resting hart rate<br>• Body weight<br>• Biorhythm<br>• Attitude toward training |
| Application of physiotherapy after workout | Meditation |
| X-training as different sport activity | Visualization |
| Lighter session(s)—within microcycle | Stationary breathing exercises |
| Lighter week(s)—within mesocycle | Relaxing music |

When high intensity training is continued for prolonged periods of time, a large amount of lactic acid is accumulated in working muscles. This process is very significant, especially in running, which utilizes interval training.

Several studies have indicated that muscular acidosis/lactate accumulation during high intensity workouts (>85% VO2 max) has significant influence on muscle fatigue and performance deterioration. In order to obtain maximum performance benefits, almost complete removal of acidosis must occur. From the research data, the maximal blood lactate concentration peak is about 20mmol/l and only rarely do athletes substantially exceed this level. Concentrations approaching this level can be generated very quickly only during maximum intensity training, mostly shorter high intensity intervals in Levels 5–6.

*Table 11: Energy system and recovery times (adapted from Recovery and Regeneration, compiled articles for the International Coaching School, Victoria, BC, Canada, 1993)*

| Energy system | Recovery time |
| --- | --- |
| ATP-PC | 2–5 minutes |
| Alactic $O_2$ (oxygen) debt | 3–5 minutes |
| $O_2$ Myoglobin | 30–60 minutes (exercise recovery) |
| Removal of lactate from muscle and blood | 60–120 minutes (rest recovery) |
| Muscle glycogen | > 46 hours |

Active rest during and immediately after interval sessions is important to flush out lactate. The removal of accumulated lactate following high intensity exercises can be accelerated by application of active recovery (Belcastro and Bonen, 1975). It has been discovered that any post-training regenerative runs have positive influence on reducing muscle's lactic acid concentration. Those two authors also have assumed that the optimal lactate reduction occurs at 32% of VO2 max or exceeds the anaerobic threshold of 3,5 to 4,5 mmol/l of lactic acid.

- Easy run with intensity about 60% of VO2 max
- Easy interval (tempo extensive) with running section from 100–300m (ex. 6x200m)

- Easy run or run combined with stride-rhythm interval on 100m distance (ex. 12x100m)
- Combination of easy run and walk

The warm-down should not exceed 12–15 minutes.

## Post-Training Regeneration Modalities

Some of the most effective modalities to accelerate regeneration post training session are:

- Hydrotherapy
- Sauna
- Sport massage
- Nutrition
- Meditation

The first three modalities for recovery work by increasing blood flow to the muscle tissue, which will help drive nutrients in the tissue and cells, then remove metabolic waste. This is effective because there is little systemic stress to the other body systems.

**Hydrotherapy**

Hydrotherapy modalities are able to significantly speed up the recovery. It is becoming the treatment of choice for fatigue from a single training session. It is effective in the acceleration of removal of lactic acid and has been effective for overtraining syndrome, injury treatment, and after early post-surgical rehabilitation.

Water therapy uses the effects of water massage, contrast bath (alternation of hot and cold water stimuli), mineral bath, and whirlpool to reduce the levels of muscle stiffness, muscle pain and soreness, and muscle spasm.

**Contrast Bath/Shower Modality**

Hydrotherapy of bath and showers is the simplest and easiest to implement. It involves the external application of warm or cold water, or alternation. The temperature of water for bath/shower range from 10C to 45C. Water treatment increases circulation of blood and decreases blood pressure by reflex of expansion or contraction of blood vessels. When blood flows freely through the athlete's body, it removes waste products of metabolism like lactic acid and carbon dioxide, and increases delivering high energy nourishment. Athletes' muscles will feel fresh, relaxed, and ready again for intensive work.

General guidance for using hydrotherapy modalities uses application of a hot/cold regimen a minimum of three times during a single treatment. The best recovery effect is achieved with alternating hot bath/shower of 35–38C with cold bath/shower of 10–16C. The duration of a single application of hot bath/shower range from 3–5 minutes where cold bath/shower lasts 30–60 seconds. The entire recovery session using contrast bath/shower must end with a warm shower. The difference between a shower and bath is that a shower can be use more frequently within a single training session, where muscles are starting to tighten up, mainly after speed and plyometric sessions.

Baths are a more robust method of regeneration. It is recommended to apply the bath a minimum of one hour after completion of the workout when the initial process of recovery is completed, and nutritional supplementation has been ingested. It is best at the end of day/final training session. After competition it is very useful to use the mineral bath using sea salt or Epsom salts . Mineral baths improve circulation in the skin and increases metabolic rates. The water temperature should be between 36C–40C and the duration is 10–20 minutes (Matuszewski (1993).

Depending on the condition of physiotherapy facilities and qualifications of staff, there are many variations of water/bath treatments:

- Pine
- Compressed air
- Vibration
- Scottish shower
- Heat chambers: 10–30% RH
- Steam baths: 90–100% RH

Another option is whirlpool treatment. The warmth of spa water, combined with the stimulation of jet massage, relaxes muscles and decreases the inflammation of the joints associated with stiffness and pain.

Benefits
- Increase circulation of body fluids
- Increase rate of metabolism
- Accelerate removal of metabolic waste (lactic acid)
- Lowering of muscle tone
- The promotion of mental relaxation

**Sauna**

The application of a sauna has effects similar to those of hydrotherapy. Sauna affects the whole body and is very intensive stimulus that increases the rate of metabolism and the circulation of the body fluids, thus aiding the removal of metabolic waste (Matuszewski, 1993).

Before treatment the athlete must be rehydrated, then take a warm shower (to moisturize the body). It is recommended to do 2–3 sauna cycles during a single session. The last sauna cycle must end with a cold shower and a minimum of 30 minutes of relaxing rest. The duration of a single sauna cycle does not last for more than 5 minutes. The best effect is when a sauna is alternated with a one-minute cold shower. The temperature of the dry sauna ranges from 60C on the lower bench to the 120–140C on the highest bench. The humidity of the air is between 5 and 15%.

Within one week, 1–3 sauna treatments can be applied. The highest number of 3 is recommended during high overload during camps, high volume, or intensity weeks.

**Pool Workouts**
Pool workouts are an effective means of rehabilitation/recovery from injury, and they allow slower movements with resistance which augments the rehabilitation process. Further, the increased compressive forces and warm temperature on joints decreases inflammation and stress, which allows activity immediately after injury. When I worked in a sports medicine clinic we would have athletes on an underwater treadmill within 24 hours of knee surgery; this accelerated the rehabilitation process with excellent long-term performance outcomes.

Moving in water is easier than moving on land due to water displacement force. It is used very effectively as a means to maintain cardiovascular fitness without the musculoskeletal stresses. Resistance loads can be increased through deep-water exercises or executed with dumbbells. The range of motion and strength of joints also increases. In the shallow water with aqua jogger unloading (to waist), technical speed workouts including skips and turnover drills can be applied.
Pool workouts will not replace the training effects of intense strength and plyometrics-speed exercising on land, but it mobilizes the athlete to make a significant effort and accelerates the progress of recovery.

**Benefits**

- Relief of pain and spasm syndromes
- Rehabilitation after injury
- Rehabilitation after surgery
- Improving overall fitness levels
- Strengthening muscles
- Improving strength and range of the motion of joints
- Maintaining and developing endurance capacity (aerobic and anaerobic)
- Maintaining technical skills
- Developing confidence
- Mobilization

**Sport Massage**

The most effective means of total restoration of training capacity after a maximal intensity training session is sport massage. Sport massage is often recognized as the method of reflex therapy. Its positive action is tied in with excitation of the nerve endings in the skin, muscle, and vessel walls that bring about reflex reactions from separate organs and from the higher brain centers. All of these organs are accompanied with increased size of the vessels, accelerated blood and lymph flow, improved blood circulation, and nourishment of the tissues.

The sport massage must be an integral portion of the sport training program and should bring positive changes in the neuro-muscular system by:

1. Decreasing fatigue of exercising muscles
2. Improving muscles' contractile ability

3. Improving the condition of impulses
4. Improving absorption of fat
5. Strengthening the breakup of protein products
6. Increasing the total body exchange of products

*Table 12: Adapted from Recovery and Regeneration, compiled articles for the International Coaching School, Victoria, BC, Canada (1993)*

| MAIN EFFECTS | MAIN ADVANTAGES |
|---|---|
| Physiological effects | |
| | 1. Increase flexibility<br>2. Increase blood flow |
| Overall result is muscle relaxation | |
| | 1. Increase oxygen/nutrients to muscle<br>2. Decrease amount of metabolic waste in muscles<br>3. Increase exchange of substances between blood and muscles' cells |
| Psychological effects | |
| | 1. Decrease stress level by:<br>• lower HR and BP<br>• lower muscle tone<br>• raise skin temperature<br>• raise mood states |

It has been known that the application of restorative massage is 2–3 times more effective than passive recovery. Restorative massage is one of the best methods of active rest. It is best applied in the following ways:

1) When there is very strong fatigue after great physical loads (plyometrics or overspeed), especially after tough competition, restorative massage should take place a minimum of 1–2 hours after end of contest. At the beginning it is light and later the massage is deeper and more energetic. The purpose of this type of massage is to decrease the activity of the excitatory process, which is increased under the influence of the physical and physiological loads.

2) The type of training phase or cycle. During the general preparation phase, when load and intensity have mostly sub-maximum character, it should be recommended to apply a lighter form of restorative massage with a duration of about 20 minutes. When the intensity and volume increases during special preparation phases, the restorative massage is extended. The extreme high intensity training mostly during pre-competition and competition phase will move the duration of massage to about 40 minutes.

3) In the competition period, and especially during the prolonged competition (first round, semifinal, finals, or tournament), we don't have enough time for maximum regeneration. In this case, restorative massage should be applied directly after the first competition. Then massage will be carried out with the goal of warming the muscles and to maintaining their work capacity. To relax the muscle stroking methods are used, which slow down muscle activity, and are recommended. The most effective include squeezing and kneading techniques that are utilized after each shaking or vibrational massage movement.

The greatest regenerative effect is from a combination of hydrotherapy and massage. This kind of treatment will accelerate and improve the exchange processes in the athlete's body.

## Nutrition: Energy and Muscle Glycogen Replenishment

A hard training session results in fatigue through a depletion of energy reserves, and tissues being broken down (a catabolic process) and causing "tissue damage." The amount of tissue damage resulting from exercises depends on the type and length of activity undertaken. Exercise in which eccentric contraction predominates (running downhill, rapid stopping, plyometrics, or strength training with free weight) causes significantly more tissue damage than purely activities with dominant character of concentric contraction. The tissue damage impairs replenishment of energy reserve (muscle glycogen and high-energy phosphate) for up to 7–10 days after a hard eccentric training session, despite complete rest and high carbohydrate intake throughout the recovery period. This indicates energy replenishment delays recovery and contributes to increasing fatigue in subsequent training sessions. In order to avoid the prolonged process of natural restoration of damaged muscle tissues we need to accelerate this process by rapid replenishment of energy fuel stores, in particular muscle and liver glycogen (Gillman ,1994).

As we know, the most important nutrient for achieving peak performance is carbohydrate. Therefore, a busy competition schedule or heavy training session (intense and long) or entire microcycle is a big challenge to carbohydrate stores.

To review, carbohydrates are divided into two categories: simple and complex. Simple carbohydrates circulate in your blood as glucose (or blood sugar). They are in the form of a single sugar unit (monosaccaraides) or as two sugar units linked together (disaccharides). The simple carbohydrates have less importance for sport because foods high in sugar are "empty calories," which means calories without added nutritional value. The energy in simple carbohydrates is realized immediately and if not consumed, it is transformed and stored as fat.

The second group of carbohydrates is complex carbohydrates. They are a chain of simple units of glucose. A more important value for sport activities has another complex carbohydrate—glycogen—that is stored as an energy reserve in the muscle and liver. Glycogen is important because the rate of energy released from complex carbohydrates is much slower, giving the body an opportunity to consume this energy source before it is converted into fat.

## Psycho-Regulatory Training

The techniques mentioned earlier belong to the active methods of restoration that involve the physical exertion of the athlete. Active rest plays an important role in the recovery process because it is necessary to apply passive methods of rest in order to regenerate the athlete psychologically. Passive rest refers to a number of processes that have a significant impact on the athlete's emotional and psychological state with high intensity training and competition. Psycho-regulatory training refers to a number of processes generally used to aid an athlete's emotional and psychological state following stresses such as:

- Breathing exercises
- Muscle relaxation techniques
- Meditation
- Floatation
- Relaxation massage
- Music
- Light therapies

The most practical and accessible methods are breathing exercises and meditation. The goal of these modalities is to decrease anxiety, regenerate your neuro-muscular system, and improve concentration—which, in turn, will improve sleep and cognitive performance.

It all starts with diaphragmatic breathing. Diaphragmatic breathing is critical to resetting and activating your core. The diaphragm, along with the transverse abdominis and pelvic floor, form the basic reflexive core. Intentional breathing using the diaphragm activates the other muscles of the reflexive core via neural and fascial connections—hence, it is the gateway into the reflexive core. Head nods and rolling help reset and stimulate your ocular-vestibular system, which is integrally related to developing proprioception and balance.

**Diaphragm Breathing**
Restores muscle proprioceptive reactivity, also shifts CNS from sympathetic to para-sympathetic (i.e., stress to rest and digest).

Lay on stomach (or back), forehead resting on flat hands, legs extended. Belly-breathe deeply in and out through your nose. Your exhale should be twice as long as your inhale. Your tongue should be pressing on the roof of your mouth just behind your teeth. On the inhale push your belly button into the ground and push it up as much as possible. The belly should always rise before the shoulders. Breathe for about 2–3 mins, then flip over on your back and hold your knees up with your hands and keep focusing on the deep breaths for another 1–2 mins.

**Meditation**
There are many different methods of meditation, and like many modalities, what will work best is an individual choice. One of the simplest methods is to start with 20 minutes of meditation once a day. Find a quiet place and sit comfortably upright, close your eyes, and focus on your breathing.

**Key Points**
- Don't meditate just before going to bed.
- Have a set routine.
- Give it time: The first 1–2 weeks you will find your thoughts running non-stop, so focus on your breathing and not the thoughts. Don't fight them, just let them go.
- Use a focusing word on your exhale to re-focus away from racing thoughts.

# 8
# Competition: Putting It All Together

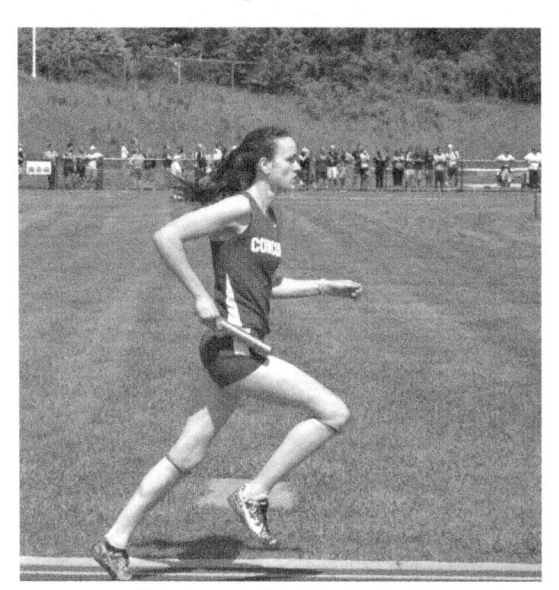

(Courtesy of Michele Andy)

*"The best-laid plans of mice and men often go awry. No matter how carefully a project is planned, something may still go wrong with it."*
—Robert Burns

So you have taken all of the above information and applied it to increase your physiological performance. However, in spite of our best preparation, sometimes what we can do in training does not translate into the race performances we expect. Below are some ideas to help you get the most out of your competitive efforts. We run fastest when we are relaxed, add some performance stress, and all of a sudden we are running a minute slower per kilometer with our heart rate 40 beats higher than in practice. This is often due to the stress and anxiety we can have with competition. We can often reduce our race anxiety with a couple of interventions. Realistic goal setting can reduce the stress we put on ourselves regarding race outcomes. A well-designed pre-race routine will help relax, focus, and prepare us physiologically for a strong race performance and diaphragmatic breathing will reduce the fight-or-flight response with the adrenaline dump we can get going into competition.

## Psychological Preparation

Psychological interventions are very useful in preparing a runner through the course of the season. With a good plan a runner will have well-defined performance goals and expectations. This will go a long way to reduce unrealistic expectations that can drive runner anxiety. On the positive side, if the runner is satisfied with reaching their goals they will be more confident and likely to continue with the sport.

### Goal Setting

Goal setting is a critical first step to having realistic competitive expectations. It is important for the coach to sit down with the athlete (or athlete plan themselves) and discuss what the athlete hopes to achieve in their season. The coach should help the athlete in defining what they plan to achieve for their short-term (fitness, technical goals), intermediate (season competitive, fitness, technical goals), and long-term (dream goals: run in college, Olympics, win world masters) goals. For each time frame there should be outcome and process goals. Outcome goals are measurable physical and competitive outcomes, such as run a 4-minute 1000-meter race for testing, qualify for state championships. Process goals are the specific training steps to achieve the outcome goal such as train 400 hours, improve technique, or core strength.

This stepwise organization will provide a clear and well-communicated plan to work synergistically with the training plan. This helps the athlete in identifying possible barriers to improving performance and their enjoyment of running. Having good feedback from the coach in goal setting will go a long way in reducing the athlete's anxiety going into the season. If the runner is new and running an average of 5:30 per kilometer pace and wants to make Junior Nationals, then it is the coach's role to help the runner plan a realistic timeline and path to achieve this goal, or even adjust the goal all together.

**Key Points**
- Start with reviewing previous season
- Set a dream goal then work backwards with realistic time frame
- Set process goals to reach dream goal
- Set intermediate and short-term goals with outcome and process sub-goals
- Sub-goals need to be specific and measurable
- Have a time frame for each goal
- Have evaluation criteria for each goal
- Determine limiting factors and barriers for each goal

## Psychological Barriers to Performance

### Race Anxiety

Anxiety is the most deleterious barrier to performing well for an athlete. This is often evidenced by an athlete running well in practice then have poor performance in races. Often athletes will become so anxious before races that they don't sleep or eat well prior to the race, and even become physically sick, due to repeated stress on their immune system. On race day the athlete is so anxious that their muscles become tight and technique suffers, hence making the runner extremely inefficient.

Many factors drive race anxiety, the most frequent one is unrealistic performance expectations. This can be mitigated to a large degree with good goal setting. One can also attempt to create training circumstances (time trials), inter-squad races, or interval sessions where each runner leads the pack, that simulate race circumstances, and the coach can assist their athletes in coping with this stress through well-structured training, pre-race routine, and relaxation exercises.

For starters remember why you are competing; hopefully competition is just one part of your path as an athlete and you are in it for the love of the process of attaining sport mastery, being fit and out in nature, or with great friends.

When I first started racing I had aspirations of turning my passion of Nordic skiing into a long-term venture, so much of how I viewed my success was based on my competitive performance. This drove a great deal of race anxiety in me and as a result my race performances were sub-optimal. Halfway through my warm-up I would feel like I was at race pace, and when I was racing I felt like no matter how hard I pushed I was not skiing much faster than I was on an easy training session. Much of this was driven by unrealistic expectations I was putting on myself. My coach in college, Cory Schwartz, saw this, and he encouraged me to race as frequently as possible for one season. He was great at relaxing me by putting the race in perspective and reminding me that this was one of many races that I would race, that the outcome of this single race will have no bearing on my overall racing career. It is your cumulative performance that matters.

Look at what thoughts are driving you to be so stressed. If it is unrealistic expectations of performance, change your timeline. On average it takes 10,000 hours of training to develop into an elite runner. If you are in high school and hoping to run in college you may need more time to develop. There is no way around this, so goals and timeline will need to be restructured.

For the physiological symptoms of anxiety (butterflies in stomach, feeling of nausea or nervous gut, increased heart rate, and feelings of nervousness), one of the best interventions is diaphragmatic breathing (see recovery section). This will shift your physiological stress response to a more calm and focused state.

The next step will be to have a well-designed pre-race routine that gets you in your optimal performance state. Every athlete performs best at slightly different physiological/psychological arousal levels. Too over-aroused (race anxiety) and you will not perform well; the same goes with being too under-aroused.

## Peaking for Competition

Peaking for competition is the point of your season where you are preparing for your best performance of the season. The process of peaking is different for every individual; based upon their age, event, level of fitness, and recovery. For newer athletes there will be some trial and error in this process as you are learning about your body and it's regenerative ability. Going into the last 7-10 days before major competitions I always say to the athletes I coach 'that your fitness is all in the bank at this point, over the next 7-10 days no training you do will significantly improve your performance, but you can certainly do too much or not rest/taper enough and have a poor performance.' This is a learned skill for many athletes. I remember at several national championship races seeing coaches running their athletes through very long intense workouts 2-3 days before competition, never did those athletes have standout performances.

Going into those last weeks of competition it is important to be developing one's peak capacity. Endurance, strength, power, anaerobic capacity have all been developed in the prior months, doing more than maintainence of these biomotor abilities during your peaking phase will lead to excessive fatigue.

**Key points**

Plan peak for competition as starting point for training plan, then work backwards

Last macrocycle should have 3 consecutive loading weeks followed by 2 unloading/recovery weeks

Unloading weeks should have 30-40% less volume with a focus on maintaining same intensity level (but 30-40% lower volume of intensity)

Do not do any long endurance workouts in the last 7-10 days

For intensity do 1-2 short intensity sessions early in the week

Older athletes require a longer unloading phase due to decreased regenerative capacity

With good peaking the athlete should feel rested, eager to compete and slightly irritable due to the decreased training load.

# Race Day

**Pre-Race Routine**

Have a set routine and timeline that works for you to get warmed up mentally and physically to be prepared as best as you can be. Eat a good meal three hours prior to racing, snack as needed to keep your energy up. Don't have any food with a high fat content in that window, it will delay your digestive transit time and your body will still be putting energy into digesting your food versus energy into a maximal physical effort. If you tend to be anxious fat will only make your digestive tract more irritable.

**Pre-Race Nutrition**

Pre-Race meal 3 hours prior to race.

- One white flour bagel and half cup active yogurt
- A banana and a cup of active yogurt
- One white flour bagel and half cup active yogurt
- Cereal or oatmeal with milk, eggs
- Oatmeal, cream of wheat, or rice
- One soy protein-enhanced pancake, sweetened with a serving of Hammer Gel

Best pre-race snacks (take on the bus with you!) are easily digestible
foods: low to high glycemic index foods. These are: Cheerios, oatmeal with
apples, pasta, breads, popcorn, bananas, oranges, yogurt. Avoid fruit juices.

Summary & pre-race meal suggestions

- Take a pre-race meal of 200–400 calories at least three hours before exercise.
- Focus on complex carbs, starches, and a little protein for your pre-race meal.
- Avoid high fiber, simple sugars, and high fat in your pre-race meal.
- If you must, take a small amount of your supplemental fuel (Hammer Gel, etc.) about five minutes before exercise.
- Make sure you re-supply your muscle glycogen by taking a good recovery meal after your workouts.

As a coach I had athletes use the following timeline to great success.

**Schedule for Race time at 1000 (10:00 am)**

**0600:** Eat breakfast
**0800:** Arrive at race venue
**0800–0830:** Eat a snack as needed
Get race bib
**0900:** Roll muscles out, do rocking and neuromuscular re-set exercises
**0930:** Start warm-up ( walk/jog course if 5k loop)
**0940:** Re-hydrate, continue warm-up**1000:** Race

**Specialized Pre-Race Warm-Up**
How you warm up has a huge impact on how fast you will race. You need to prime the pump to get your body ready to push hard right out of the gate. For junior-level runners where you race 5k this is all the more important. Research has shown that if you do a progressive warm-up, and spend time at race pace, you will be able to race faster than if you had a lower intensity warm-up. Logically many athletes think that if they get into race pace they will not have the energy to be fast in the race. BUT that is not how the human body works. We have to stress it at race pace

so it is firing on all cylinders to race full-throttle right from the start and maintain a sustained high pace. Your lactate buffering capacity will be more effective if you have switched gears into this higher intensity mode prior to the race.

**Pre-Race Warm-Up**

Start 20–30 minutes prior to the race depending on the race format. Stay hydrated during your warm-up; have a water bottle with you to drink over these 20–30 minutes.

- Level 1 run: 5 minutes
- Level 2 run: 5 minutes
- Level 3 run: 2–3 minutes
- Level 4 run: 4 minutes
- 2 minutes rest, 55/5s for 3–5 minutes
- Strip down and go to start line

**Warm-Down**

Immediately after your race, get warm clothes on, grab your water bottle, rehydrate, and start running in Level 1 for 5 minutes, then run at Level 3 for 4–7 minutes, then finish with Level 1 for 3–5 minutes. Research has found that recovery from races is much more effective when the runner's post-race warm-down includes 4–7 minutes in Level 3 to flush metabolic waste. This is even more critical if you are racing on consecutive days. After your warm-down drink Hammer Recoverite and change into warm clothes.

Hot-wash after the race: speak with your coach and evaluate what did and did not go well. Be honest with yourself, take responsibility for what you can improve upon, and integrate these changes into your training and next race. Every race is a learning process…it takes years to figure out what works best for you.

The information in this book will hopefully go a long way for you to plan and organize your training to a higher level!

# Acknowledgements

This book would not have been possible without the inspiration of my family who have encouraged me to put years of thoughts and experiences on paper. Help editing and clarifying thoughts on Original Strength and other training concepts would not have been possible without Mark Shropshire's expertise and wisdom. Lastly many thanks to my coach and good friend Krzysztof Mackala, who has been a mentor, and encouraged me (and many others) to pursue coaching, and learn about advanced, applied concepts of sports training that have led to cutting edge methods of developing athletes to their peak potential.

# About the Author

Stuart Kremzner is the CEO of E3 Sports Performance. He has been coaching/training athletes for 25 years and trained over 300 elite and professional athletes (NFL, NHL, NBA), as well as elite military and federal law enforcement groups.

Professionally, Stuart directed and started up several of the nation's premier sports training and sports medicine facilities in Utah and Illinois. During his tenure there he trained elite Olympic, professional, college, junior-level, and master-level athletes. In addition he was on the faculty at Weber State University where he taught exercise science. Stuart worked closely with the WSU coaches developing training programs for the WSU Track and Field, Soccer, Basketball, and Volleyball, teams. The WSU Men's and Women's Basketball teams qualified for the 2003 NCAA Championships (women for 2004 as well).

Stuart has coached and raced throughout his career. For running he has worked with US Olympic Marathon runners, Triathletes, top ranked master Ultra-marathon runners, elite junior track and X-C athletes. He has coached high school track and master's running camps and clinics as well. Stuart earned his Master's in Exercise Physiology at University of Montana, and has certifications as NSCA CSCS, FMS Level II, Original Strength and USSA level 200 coach.

# References

Aalberg, J. Modern Endurance Training, Fasterskier Article 2002.

Abe, D., Sakaguchi, Y., Tsuchimochi, H., Endo, M., Miyake, K., Miyahiro, S., ... & Niihata, S. (1999). Assessment of long-distance running performance in elite male runners using onset of blood lactate accumulation. *Applied human science: journal of physiological anthropology*, *18*(2), 25-29.

Anderson, T., Morton, C., Shropshire, M., (2018). *Original Strength Performance: The Next Level*. OS Press.

Anderson, T., Neupert, G., (2013). *Original Strength*. OS Press.

Anderson, T., Neupert, G., (2018). Pressing Reset: *Original Strength Reloaded*. OS Press.

Barnes, K. R., & Kilding, A. E. (2015). Running economy: measurement, norms, and determining factors. *Sports medicine-open*, *1*(1), 1-15.

Belcastro, A. N., & Bonen, A. (1975). Lactic acid removal rates during controlled and uncontrolled recovery exercise. *Journal of applied physiology*, *39*(6), 932-936.

Boyle, M. (2007). Joint by Joint Approach to Training. *T Nation, LLC*.

Calder, A. (2007). *Recovery and Regeneration for Long-Term Athlete Development*. Canadian Sport Centres.

Calder, A. (2004). Recovery and regeneration. *FHS-LEEDS-*, 12-15.

Calder, A. (1990). Restoration and Regeneration as Essential Components within Training Programs. *Excel*, *6*(3), 15-19.

Cook, G. (2010). *Movement: Functional movement systems: Screening, assessment, corrective strategies*. On Target Publications.

Daniels, J. (2005). *Daniels' running formula [proven programs 800 m to the marathon]*. Human Kinetics.

Drabik, J. (1996). Children and sports training. *Island Point, VT: Stadion Publishing Company*.

Dubois, B., Esculier, J. F., Frémont, P., Moore, L., & Richards, C. (2015). Effects of minimalist and traditional running shoes on injury rates: a pilot randomised controlled trial. *Footwear Science*, *7*(3), 159-164.

Enoksen, E., Tjelta, A. R., & Tjelta, L. I. (2011). Distribution of training volume and intensity of elite male and female track and marathon runners. *International Journal of Sports Science & Coaching*, 6(2), 273-293.

Faiss, R., Willis, S., Born, D. P., Sperlich, B., Vesin, J. M., Holmberg, H. C., & Millet, G. P. (2015). Repeated double-poling sprint training in hypoxia by competitive cross-country runners. *Medicine and science in sports and exercise*, 47(4), 809-817.

Gillam, I. Monitoring the athlete recovery in training, High Performance Coaching Seminar on Recovery, Department of Human Movement Science, RMIT, Budoora Campus.

Goss, D. L., Lewek, M., Yu, B., Ware, W. B., Teyhen, D. S., & Gross, M. T. (2015). Lower extremity biomechanics and self-reported foot-strike patterns among runners in traditional and minimalist shoes. *Journal of athletic training*, 50(6), 603-611.

Grandjean & Ruud. (1994). Nutrition for Cyclists, Clinics in Sports Med. Vol 13(1);235-246. Jan 1994.

Grandjean, A & Rudd, JS (1994) Energy intake of athletes. In Oxford Textbook of Sports Medicine, pp. 53–65 [Harries, M, Williams, C, Stanish, WD and Micheli, LJ, editors] Oxford: Oxford University Press.

Hanlon, T. (1987). Injuries in runners: Lysholm J, Wiklander J Am J Sports Med 15: 168–171 Jun 1987. *Annals of Emergency Medicine*, 16(12), 1404.

Holmberg, H. C. (2015). The elite cross-country runner provides unique insights into human exercise physiology. *Scandinavian journal of medicine & science in sports*, 25, 100-109.

Helgerud, J., Høydal, K., Wang, E., Karlsen, T., Berg, P., Bjerkaas, M, & Hoff, J. (2007). Aerobic high-intensity intervals improve V̇O2max more than moderate training. *Medicine & Science in Sports & Exercise, 39*(4), 665-671.

Heggelund, J., Fimland, M. S., Helgerud, J. & Hoff, J. (2013). Maximal strength training improves work economy, rate of force development and maximal strength more than conventional strength training. *European journal of applied physiology, 113*(6), 1565-1573.

Hoff, J., Helgerud, J., & Wisloeff, U. L. R. I. K. (1999). Maximal strength training improves work economy in trained female cross-country runners. *Medicine and science in sports and exercise, 31*(6), 870-877.

Hoffman-Goetz, L. & Pedersen, B. K. (1994). Exercise and the immune system: A model of the stress response? *Immunology Today, 15*(8), 382-387.

Hooper, S. L., Mackinnon, L. T., Gordon, R. D., & Bachmann, A. W. (1993). Hormonal responses of elite swimmers to overtraining. *Medicine and science in sports and exercise, 25*(6), 741-747.

(Iaia, & Bangsbo, 2010). Skovgaard, C., Almquist, N. W., & Bangsbo, J. (2018). The effect of repeated periods of speed endurance training on performance, running economy, and muscle adaptations. *Scandinavian journal of medicine & science in sports, 28*(2), 381-390.

Iaia, F., & Bangsbo, J. (2010). Speed endurance training is a powerful stimulus for physiological adaptations and performance improvements of athletes. *Scandinavian journal of medicine & science in sports, 20*, 11-23.

Kanaley, J. A., & Hartman, M. L. (2002). Cortisol and growth hormone responses to exercise. *The Endocrinologist*, *12*(5), 421-432.

Karlsen, T, and Aalberg, J. (2004). The Art of Interval Training: A discussion on how long each interval should be, how many sessions per week you should do and what the total length of each session should be. Fasterskier Article.

Komi, P. V., Ito, A., Sjödin, B., Wallenstein, R., & Karlsson, J. (1981). Muscle metabolism, lactate breaking point, and biomechanical features of endurance running. *International journal of sports medicine*, *2*(03), 148-153.

Krestovnikov, A. N. (1951). Essays on the Physiology of Physical Exercises. *Moscow: Fizkultura i sport*.

Laursen, Paul & Jenkins, David. (2002). The scientific basis for high-intensity interval training: Optimising training programmes and maximising performance in highly trained endurance athletes. Sports medicine (Auckland, N.Z.). 32. 53-73.

Lieberman, D. E., Venkadesan, M., Werbel, W. A., Daoud, A. I., D'andrea, S., Davis, I. S., ... & Pitsiladis, Y. (2010). Foot strike patterns and collision forces in habitually barefoot versus shod runners. *Nature*, *463*(7280), 531-535.

Lieberman, D. E., Warrener, A. G., Wang, J., & Castillo, E. R. (2015). Effects of stride frequency and foot position at landing on braking force, hip torque, impact peak force and the metabolic cost of running in humans. *Journal of Experimental Biology*, *218*(21), 3406-3414.

Loko, J., Sikkut, T., & Aule, R. (1996). Sensitive periods in physical development. *Modern Athlete and Coach*, *34*(2), 26-29.

Mackala, K., Fostiak, M., Schweyen, B., Osik, T., & Coch, M. (2019). Acute Effects of a Speed Training Program on Sprinting Step Kinematics and Performance. *International journal of environmental research and public health, 16*(17), 3138.

Marti, B., Vader, J. P., Minder, C. E., & Abelin, T. (1988). On the epidemiology of running injuries: the 1984 Bern Grand-Prix study. *The American Journal of Sports Medicine, 16*(3), 285-294.

Matuszewski, W. (1992). The role of regeneration in sport, in The Charlie Francis training system
(ed. Francis C. and Patterson P.) TBLI Publications Inc. 1992.

McDougall, C. (2010). *Born to run: The hidden tribe, the ultra-runners, and the greatest race the world has never seen.* Profile Books.

Milner, C. E., Ferber, R., Pollard, C. D., Hamill, J. O. S. E. P. H., & Davis, I. S. (2006). Biomechanical factors associated with tibial stress fracture in female runners. *Medicine & Science in Sports & Exercise, 38*(2), 323-328.

Moore, I. S. (2016). Is there an economical running technique? A review of modifiable biomechanical factors affecting running economy. *Sports Medicine, 46*(6), 793-807.

Morgan, D. W., Martin, P. E., & Krahenbuhl, G. S. (1989). Factors affecting running economy. *Sports Med, 7*(5), 310-330.

Mroczek, D., Mackala, K., Chmura, P., Superlak, E., Konefal, M., Seweryniak, T., ... & Chmura, J. (2019). Effects of Plyometrics Training on Muscle Stiffness Changes in Male Volleyball Players. The Journal of Strength & Conditioning Research, 33(4), 910-921.

Myers, T. W. (2013). *Anatomy trains e-book: myofascial meridians for manual and movement therapists*. Elsevier Health Sciences.

Napier, C., MacLean, C. L., Maurer, J., Taunton, J. E., & Hunt, M. A. (2019). Kinematic correlates of kinetic outcomes associated with running-related injury. *Journal of applied biomechanics*, *35*(2), 123-130.

Niemelä, M., Kulmala, J. P., Kauppi, J. P., Kosonen, J., & Äyrämö, S. (2017). Prediction of active peak force using a multilayer perceptron. *Sports Engineering*, *20*(3), 213-219.

Noehren, B., Pohl, M. B., Sanchez, Z., Cunningham, T., & Lattermann, C. (2012). Proximal and distal kinematics in female runners with patellofemoral pain. *Clinical biomechanics*, *27*(4), 366-371.

Noehren, B., Schmitz, A., Hempel, R., Westlake, C., & Black, W. (2014). Assessment of strength, flexibility, and running mechanics in men with iliotibial band syndrome. *journal of orthopaedic & sports physical therapy*, *44*(3), 217-222.

Paavolainen, L., Hakkinen, K., Hamalainen, I., Nummela, A., & Rusko, H. (1999). Explosive-strength training improves 5-km running time by improving running economy and muscle power. *Journal of applied physiology*, *86*(5), 1527-1533.

Paikov, V. B. (1985). Means of restoration in the training of speed skaters. *Soviet Sports Review*, *20*, 9-12.

Preece, S. J., Mason, D., & Bramah, C. (2016). How do elite endurance runners alter movements of the spine and pelvis as running speed increases?. *Gait & posture*, *46*, 132-134.

Richards, C. E., Magin, P. J., & Callister, R. (2009). Is your prescription of distance running shoes evidence-based?. *British journal of sports medicine, 43*(3), 159-162.

Ridge, S. T., Standifird, T., Rivera, J., Johnson, A. W., Mitchell, U., & Hunter, I. (2015). The effect of training in minimalist running shoes on running economy. *Journal of sports science & medicine, 14*(3), 643.

Santos-Concejero, J., Tam, N., Granados, C., Irazusta, J., Bidaurrazaga-Letona, I., Zabala-Lili, J., & Gil, S. M. (2014). Stride angle as a novel indicator of running economy in well-trained runners. *The Journal of Strength & Conditioning Research, 28*(7), 1889-1895.

Saunders, P. U., Telford, R. D., Pyne, D. B., Peltola, E. M., Cunningham, R. B., Gore, C. J., & Hawley, J. A. (2006). Short-term plyometric training improves running economy in highly trained middle and long distance runners. *Journal of Strength and Conditioning Research, 20*(4), 947.

Shephard, R. J., & Astrand, P. O. (Eds.). (2008). *Endurance in sport* (Vol. 2). John Wiley & Sons.

Shropshire, M. (2020) Correspondence regarding injury risk and Original Strength.

Storen, O., Helgerud, J. A. N., Stoa, E. M., & Hoff, J. A. N. (2008). Maximal strength training improves running economy in distance runners. *Medicine and science in sports and exercise, 40*(6), 1087.

Souza, R. B. (2016). An evidence-based videotaped running biomechanics analysis. *Physical medicine and rehabilitation clinics, 27*(1), 217-236.

Svedenhag, J., & Sjödin, B. (1984). Maximal and submaximal oxygen uptakes and blood lactate levels in elite male middle-and long-distance runners. *International journal of sports medicine*, *5*(05), 255-261.

Taunton, J. E., Ryan, M. B., Clement, D. B., McKenzie, D. C., Lloyd-Smith, D. R., & Zumbo, B. D. (2002). A retrospective case-control analysis of 2002 running injuries. *British journal of sports medicine*, *36*(2), 95-101.

Tjelta, L. I. (2016). The training of international level distance runners. *International Journal of Sports Science & Coaching*, *11*(1), 122-134.

Viru, A. A., & Viru, M. (2001). *Biochemical monitoring of sport training*. Human Kinetics.

Viru, A., & Viru, M. (1993). The specific nature of training on muscle: a review. *Research in Sports Medicine: An International Journal*, *4*(2), 79-98.

Viru, A., Loko, J., Harro, M., Volver, A., Laaneots, L. & Viru, M. (1999). Critical periods in the development of performance capacity during childhood and adolescence. *European Journal of Physical Education*, *4*(1), 75-119.

Yessis, M. (1982). Restoration Or Increasing the Ability to Do More Voluminous and Higher Intensity Workouts. *Strength & Conditioning Journal*, *4*(3), 38-41.

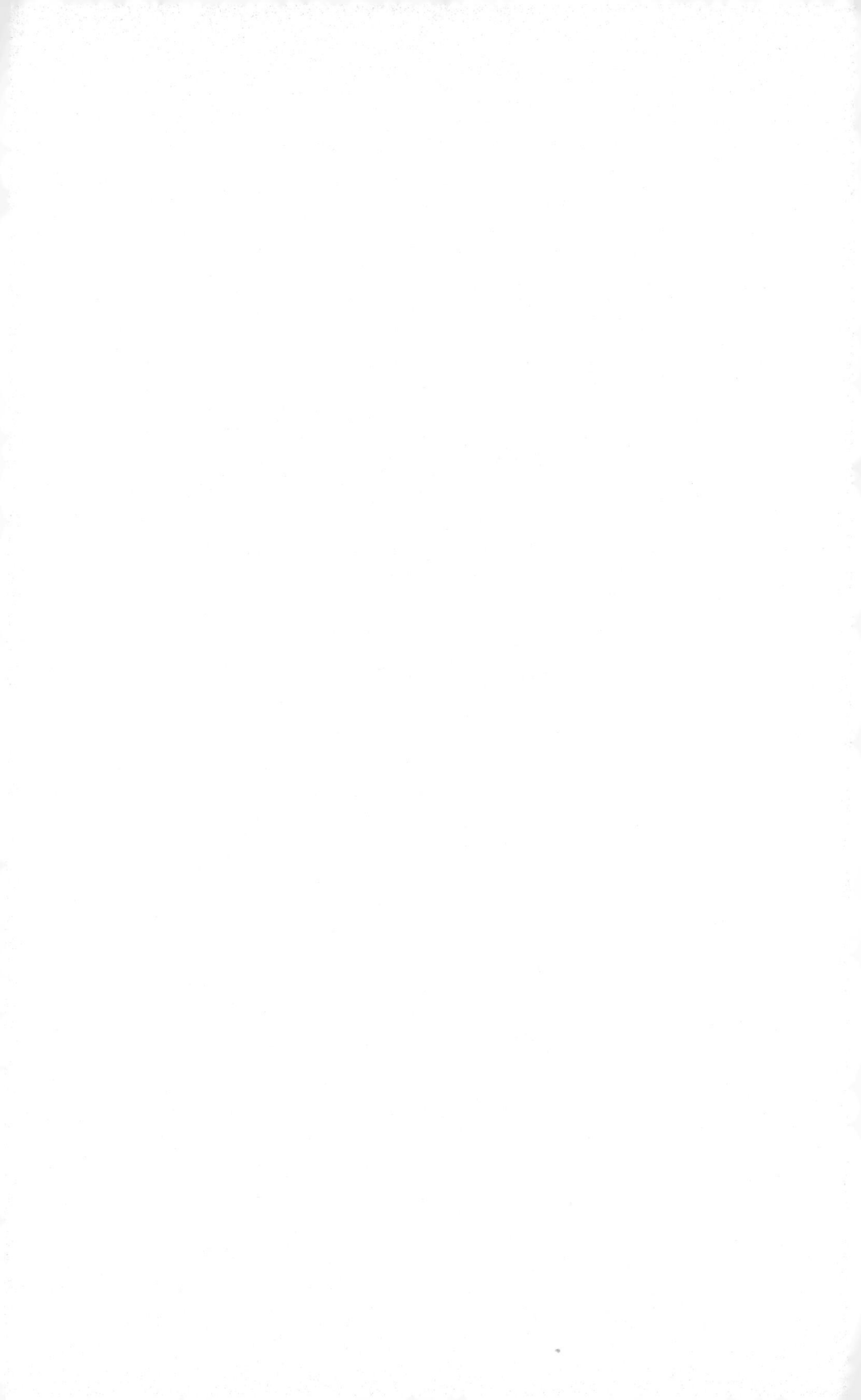

Made in the USA
Monee, IL
15 December 2020